Teaching Students in Clinical Settings

FORTHCOMING TITLES

Research Methods for Therapists
Avril Drummond

Group Work in Occupational Therapy
Linda Finlay

Stroke: Recovery and Rehabilitation
Polly Laidler

Caring for the Neurologically Damaged Adult
Ruth Nieuwenhuis

HIV and Aids Care
S. Singh and L. Cusack

Speech and Language Disorders in Children
Dilys A. Treharne

Spinal Cord Rehabilitation
Karen Whalley-Hammell

THERAPY IN PRACTICE SERIES

Edited by Jo Campling

This series of books is aimed at 'therapists' concerned with rehabilitation in a very broad sense. The intended audience particularly includes occupational therapists, physiotherapists and speech and language therapists, but many titles will also be of interest to nurses, psychologists, medical staff, social workers, teachers or volunteer workers. Some volumes are interdisciplinary, others are aimed at one particular profession. All titles will be comprehensive but concise, and practical but with due reference to relevant theory and evidence. They are not research monographs but focus on professional practice, and will be of value to both students and qualified personnel.

Teaching Students in Clinical Settings

Jackie Stengelhofen

Lecturer and Consultant in the education of health professionals and
in Speech and Language Pathology

CHAPMAN & HALL

London · Glasgow · New York · Tokyo · Melbourne · Madras

Published by Chapman & Hall, 2–6 Boundary Row, London SE1 8HN

Chapman & Hall, 2–6 Boundary Row, London SE1 8HN, UK

Blackie Academic & Professional, Wester Cleddens Road, Bishopbriggs, Glasgow G64 2NZ, UK

Chapman & Hall, 29 West 35th Street, New York NY10001, USA

Chapman & Hall Japan, Thomson Publishing Japan, Hirakawacho Nemoto Building, 6F, 1–7–11 Hirakawa-cho, Chiyoda-ku, Tokyo 102, Japan

Chapman & Hall Australia, Thomas Nelson Australia, 102 Dodds Street, South Melbourne, Victoria 3205, Australia

Chapman & Hall India, R. Seshadri, 32 Second Main Road, CIT East, Madras 600 035, India

Distributed in the USA and Canada by Singular Publishing Group Inc., 4284 41st Street, San Diego, California 92105

First edition 1993

© 1993 Jackie Stengelhofen

Typeset in 10/12 Times by Mews Photosetting, Beckenham, Kent
Printed in Great Britain by TJ Press (Padstow) Ltd, Padstow, Cornwall

ISBN 0 412 45250 2   1 56593 119 X (USA)

∞ Printed on permanent acid-free text paper, manufactured in accordance with the proposed ANSI/NISO Z 39.48-199X and ANSI Z 39.48-1984

For friends and colleagues in teaching, both in educational institutions and clinical settings. In particular to Sandra Rowan for her wisdom and support over many years, and to the students with whom we have had the privilege to work.

Contents

Contributors

Jenny Eastwood, Principal Lecturer, School of Speech Pathology,
De Montfort University

Peter Richards, Head of School of Postgraduate Studies,
Faculty of Health and Social Sciences,
University of Central England, in Birmingham

Jane Whitehouse, Speech and Language Therapist, Nunnery Wood
Language Unit, Worcester and District Health Authority

Acknowledgements

The material for this book has been developed mainly over the past 3 years, in response to the needs of health professionals attending clinical teaching courses. The efficacy of the teaching of students during periods of clinical placements takes on particular importance in the context of quality assurance. During this time it has been possible to share ideas with colleagues from many fields. It has been a rewarding experience to gather together the richness of experience from clinicians attending these courses. Many gave their ideas generously and encouraged me to continue with the preparation of this book. Where possible the specific source of examples has been given in the text. As this has not always been possible I would like to acknowledge the help and support received from clinical teachers during courses in Dudley, Hounslow and Spelthorne, Southampton and South East Hampshire, Swindon, North and South Warwickshire, and Yorkshire Region as well as the clinical teachers for the BSc Podiatry, and clinical colleages on the BSc Health Studies courses at Birmingham Polytechnic.

During the preparation of the book colleagues have given of their help most generously in commenting on a number of chapters; particular thanks are due to Carolyn Leach, orthoptist; Celia Firmin, dietitian; Thelma Harvey, physiotherapist; Linda Finlay, occupational therapist; and to Beryl Kellow, speech and language therapist, for her comments on the chapter on management skills.

A special thanks to Cath McMaster who was the first district manager to have the courage and vision to mount a multiprofessional course on clinical teaching. It was a stimulating experience which encouraged me to mount further courses and to prepare this book.

I want to thank especially the three contributors; Jenny Eastwood, Peter Richards and Jane Whitehouse, for their support, encouragement and patience, as well as for their excellent contributions.

Special thanks to Val Dinning who, in many ways, has helped me to the end, and who painstakingly read the final stages of the manuscript.

Preface

As part of the pre-registration education for students who intend to enter health care work, periods of work experience are built into the curriculum. Students are placed in work settings, generally termed clinical settings, for specified periods, ranging from single days to extended periods of time. During these placements the students are 'supervised' by qualified staff whose first responsibility is to the care of patients. It is therefore important that provision is made to support these clinicians in their role of teaching and supervising students.

Initiatives have therefore been taken to enhance clinicians' knowledge and skills in the teaching process. The principles and procedures to be used in the supervision and teaching of students are generic in nature and therefore applicable to a number of fields. This book has been prepared for use by a wide range of professionals in health fields. There is particular attention to chiropody/podiatry, dietetics, occupational therapy, orthoptics, physiotherapy, speech and language therapy and radiography, although the principles covered are also applicable to a wider spectrum of professions. The content draws on the experience of clinicians and teachers and will, it is hoped, help to disseminate the good practice which already exists.

The aims of the book are: to examine the nature and value of supervised work experience in a number of different fields; to familiarize the reader with concepts related to the curriculum; to examine the roles and responsibilities of the clinical teacher; to consider a range of teaching methods and examine their appropriateness to teaching in clinical settings; to examine how receiving departments can prepare themselves for working with students; to consider ways of helping students to become independent in their learning; to consider ways of introducing management skills to students; to examine the nature of and the ways of providing feedback to students; and to examine the methods and difficulties of the assessment of practical work and its relationship to professional competence.

The value of a multiprofessional book on the topic of clinical teaching is that it is, for the most part, free from the content of the particular fields for which students are preparing. Thus, it allows the reader to concentrate on the principles of teaching and learning being discussed, rather than being concerned about, for example, the nature of the condition being treated, the appropriateness of treatment, etc., which are the paramount daily concerns of clinicians. At points in the text the reader is encouraged to apply the ideas explored, to their own field, through specific examples, and then to generate similar examples of their own. Such examples and other practical ideas are 'boxed' in the text, in order that they can be quickly retrieved. Furthermore, in order to encourage this application, Chapters 1–8 include practical suggestions for follow-up activities.

In the first chapter, a model of professional practice is considered. Courses designed for students who are preparing for professional work are discussed in relation to the consequences the design may have on both teachers and learners. Concepts of theory and practice are considered; the model adopted is one which views theory and practice as a continuum, with the thinking nature of practice being viewed as of major importance. The teaching of theory and practice cannot, therefore, be seen as separate; this has major implications for course design and student learning. The second chapter examines methods of teaching in general and, more specifically, the methods which might be applicable to clinical teaching. Careful consideration is given to the clinic as an environment for teaching and learning. Chapter 3 explores the role of the clinical teacher. At this point the reader is ready to consider in detail ways of becoming prepared to receive a student into their department or service, in Chapter 4. An awareness of student anxieties and expectations is encouraged. As part of the preparation for working with students, teaching and learning styles and the interpersonal aspects of the teacher–student interaction are considered.

Chapter 5 concentrates on procedures to be used while the student is on placement. There is an examination of such aspects as, developing observation skills, teaching procedures and helping students to fit into the team. Chapter 6 concentrates on introducing students to management skills; this is seen as an essential part of professional practice and it is therefore important for the clinical teacher to heighten the student's awareness of management procedures.

In Chapter 7 the important area of formative feedback is fully explored. This is seen within the context of helping students to become independent practitioners who are able to evaluate their own practice. The chapter also includes an examination of the feedback which may take place when college tutors visit students on placement. The nature, content and potential difficulties of such visits are thoroughly considered. Following on from the chapter on feedback, which is a formative process, the reader is taken on to summative assessment of clinical competence. The final chapter consists of a literature review on supervised work experience, thus placing the book within a firm theoretical and research background as well as providing an introduction to the research literature for those readers who wish to explore the topic further. It also enables all readers to see the subject of clinical teaching in a wider academic and educational context.

Jackie Stengelhofen

in nature, length and status. In the UK, the College of Occupational Therapists has a well-developed sequential programme (Box 1.1). While in Dietetics, where students spend 31 weeks in placement, a range of opportunities are planned for clinicians (Box. 1.2).

Box 1.1 A sequential approach to clinical education. Adapted from information from the Post-registration Studies Committee, College of Occupational Therapists UK (1989)

---

1. **Role of clinical education;** appreciation of basic education theory. Awareness of sources of information available to students. Understanding the learning objectives at each stage of training and the need to identify the specific requirements of individual students.

2. **Planning and implementing clinical education;** planning and organizing field work within the supervisor's own clinical environment. Recognizing and responding to needs and changes. Teaching and assessment techniques. Evaluation and non-performance.

3. **Management of learning;** recognizing different ways in which attitudes, cognitive and practical skills can be acquired. Applying selected techniques to improve this understanding and performance of students and staff. Assessment of students' performance.

4. **Professional development;** developing and evaluating opportunities for learning. Observing self and others' progress and relating strategies and outcomes to theories of learning and education. Planning programmes for individual student's using a variety of settings and resources.

5. **Curriculum design;** being sufficiently familiar with professional knowledge and skill, with education theory and the needs of students, so that the supervisors can design curricula for professional education at different levels.

6. **Research and evaluation;** skilled, continuing observation of learning taking place in a variety of settings. Analysis of strategies and outcome leading to structures of controlled innovation.

There is clearly a need for constant dialogue between the college course placing students and the receiving agency. Indeed, clinicians often feel that there is not sufficient contact. Perhaps the interface between college tutors and clinicians should focus on the particular course needs and the students, and the principles of teaching and learning should be left for another forum. The author has found considerable value in offering clinical teaching courses

Box 1.2 Model for clinical supervisors' education in dietetics. British Dietetics Association UK (1990)

Ongoing education inputs	Formal clinical 'supervisors' courses	Work input
BDA trainers/tutors' meetings/study/ workshops	Pre-registration Education relevant to clinical supervision	Newly qualified; clinical areas related to supervision
'BDA Education Group' study days/workshops		With student dieticians developing clinical supervisor role
BDA study conferences	BDA clinical supervisors course 'Tier I'	
BDA specialist groups study days workshops, courses		Increased student involvement, assessment, planning
Non-BDA-relevant courses, e.g. counselling skills, training, communication training, counselling certificate, teaching certificate management courses	BDA clinical supervisors course 'Tier II' BDA Certificate for clinical tutors	Increased need for wider approach: research and evaluation

on a multiprofessional basis (Stengelhofen, 1990a). This kind of provision has the advantage of bringing health professionals together to share an area of common concern, and it discourages practitioners from focusing too much on their own field instead of the principles of teaching and learning. Furthermore, the opportunity to examine clinical teaching practices in other spheres illuminates and enhances our own often rather blinkered approaches. Having to explain to another professional what we really do in our jobs covertly improves our skills as teachers, as well as adding to our skills as team members.

It is hoped that this book will demonstrate further that the knowledge and skills to be used in clinical teaching have relevance to all fields. A rational way forward might be not to bring all the professions together for courses on clinical teaching, but to divide the professions into two groups (Stengelhofen, 1990b). Although there are common needs for students in all fields, there are some differences according to the way the groups carry out their clinical activity (Ellis, 1980, 1988). All health professionals **care about and cater for the needs of others**, but some groups do this more by technical means and others do it primarily through the interpersonal medium. Ellis avoids the terms 'helping and caring' because they are loaded, and adopts the term 'interpersonal professions' as value free. It is for each field to decide where they lie on the technical–interpersonal continuum; clearly, all fields contain both aspects. All the fields are included in this book, but some ideas presented may be more relevant to teaching students in some fields than others. Dickson and Maxwell (1985) explored this in the context of the training of physiotherapists, stressing that everything is channelled through the inter-personal medium in physiotherapy practice. It is possible that the way we work may have a major influence on the way we teach students, both in the classroom and in the clinic.

THE LITERATURE AVAILABLE ON CLINICAL TEACHING

Some professional groups, such as medics and social workers, show that they have paid considerable attention to the needs of students learning in the work place; this is indicated in the literature. Some professions publish journals solely related to education in their own fields. Readers may find the following journals of interest:

- *Medical Education*
- *Medical Teacher*
- *Education in Social Work*
- *Journal of the Association of Chiropody Teachers in the UK*

The Clinical Supervisor includes articles on all fields in health care. Articles in education journals such as:

- *Journal of Further and Higher Education*
- *Journal of the Society of Research into Higher Education*
- *Programmed Learning and Educational Technology*

will be found of value in the examination of educational principles which can be applied to teaching and learning in clinical settings.

The final chapter of this book looks more widely at some of the research literature on the value of 'supervised work experience' in the preparation of professionals. It is hoped that it will serve as a starting point for those clinical teachers who wish to extend their interests further on the topic. Some readers may find that they prefer to read Chapter 9 first, in order to set the topic of clinical teaching in its broadest context, as well as within a firm research background. Others may prefer to get on more quickly with the ideas on working with students in clinic, explored in the earlier chapters.

THE NATURE OF THEORY AND PRACTICE

Placing appropriate importance on the role of the clinician receiving the student for work experience should stem from the course team's views about the status of practice in the student's learning experience as a whole. This view needs to be upheld by validating bodies, both professional and academic. The design of some courses unfortunately suggests that 'practice' is viewed as an added extra and possibly of lower status than that which is studied in college and termed 'theory'. An alternative view is to see practice as central and the pinnacle of academic achievement, as it requires the highest level of intellectual functioning namely:

- Synthesis
- Application
- Evaluation

Bloom, 1954

Colleagues sometimes say 'she's not very bright, but she's a very good therapist'. I am always puzzled as to what exactly this can mean. The converse has been found in research in medical education which suggests that good academic performance does not necessarily imply good practice. Nevertheless adequate academic performance must be a prerequisite for competent clinical practice. Academic achievement and clinical competence must be closely related, because the large part of what clinicians do is academic, the jobs require thought, not just the carrying out of techniques and procedures. Yes, we all have high level skills which we use frequently, but much of what others can observe us doing, on the surface, appears comparatively simple. For example, counselling in dietetics, eliciting a language sample in speech and language therapy, teaching a hemiplegic to walk in physiotherapy, helping someone to dress in occupational therapy, strapping in chiropody, or taking a chest X-ray in radiography do not appear too difficult to the onlooker.

The activity itself is not the most difficult part, although we know that there are in fact many difficulties in carrying out these tasks. Students know all too well that some tasks which look incredibly easy when carried out by the experienced clinician, are a minefield for the learner. Nonetheless what is the most difficult for the practitioner is what goes on in the head;

observing and analysing the patient's problem, deciding what has to be done and evaluating the effectiveness of what has been done. The thinking part of the job is essential in the identification of the patient's needs and the provision of appropriate care. These points about what we do on the surface and what we think about while we're doing it leads us to the central issue of the relationship between the knowledge base of competence and what we actually do on the job or the nature of 'theory and practice'.

In considering the nature of theory and practice I have found it helpful to look at the literature in other professional spheres. The definitions by Schwab (1969, 1971) from education are particularly illuminating. He defines practice as:

'The discipline concerned with choice and action, in contrast with theoretic which is concerned with knowledge'.

and

'The practical is always marked by particularity the theoretical by generality'.

I especially like this second definition because of the alliteration which resonates in the health care context:

- Practical
- Particular
- Patients

So, in Schwab's terms, the theoretic is about that which is generally true, while the practical is about particular examples of the general. Schwab also talks about the 'arts of the eclectic', that is, what can be chosen from the generality of theory of a subject or discipline or even schools within these disciplines. For example, professional groups which make considerable use of psychology, will be aware of the different schools of thought and consequently the choices which have to be made from the knowledge base and the consequent differing approaches. Choices and decision-making are a central part of professional practice; experienced clinicians will be aware how frequently choice has to be made.

The first follow-up activity at the end of this chapter is on making choices. It is the major activity of health care professional to decide both the nature of a problem and the appropriate management. This discussion therefore suggests that theory and practice should not be viewed as separate but should be seen as a continuum. At one end theory attempting to solve problems or explain by seeking knowledge, at the other end practice, trying to bring about change through action. In this view theory and practice become complementary parts of the same process. This is surely what is involved in the work of all health care professionals.

Argyris and Schon (1974) take these ideas further in their work *Theory in Practice: increasing professional effectiveness*. They propose a model of practice under the title 'theories-of-action'. This has two components; (i) espoused theory, that is what we say we do, the values and strategies we proclaim publicly; (ii) 'theories-in-use', that is, what we actually do in reality. These two components may or may not be compatible. This model is helpful as it includes the possibility of the individual talking about theory, as though it will be used in practice, but not applying it. In the context of professional education this concept is particularly useful. I am sure we can all remember students who have been able to *tell* us all about it!

Argyris and Schon stress that learning to become competent in professional practice **'does not consist of learning to recite a theory; the theory-of-action has not been learned in the most important sense unless it can be put into practice'**. Furthermore they stress that theory-in-use needs to be individually created by each practitioner through his own experience. This underlines the importance of every student having enough first hand work experience, during their pre-registration course, to develop their individual theory-in-use. This view that 'theory-in-use' has to be individually created in professional preparation means that work experience, i.e. that which is usually termed the practical and is largely learnt through clinical practice, must be placed centrally in the curriculum.

Curriculum developers presumably believe that the overall design of a course and the syllabus content have a direct bearing on the preparation of students for practice. At the centre of this is the need to enable students not only to acquire knowledge and skills and appropriate attitudes, but to be able to apply these competently in the exercise of their profession. There are therefore two major questions for professionals to ask:
1.   What is the reality of professional practice?
2.   How does the course of study prepare the student for this reality?

TEACHERS' RESPONSIBILITIES

The term 'espoused theory' used by Argyris and Schon, is a reminder that college-based teachers need to be constantly vigilant, in that although they have a responsiblity to introduce students to the latest research findings, these should not be so far removed from the reality of the working situation that it is impossible for students to apply them in their clinical practice. Conversely, teachers have a responsiblity to include in their classroom teaching current clinical practices which, in fact, may be ahead in the field, for indeed it is often practice which informs theory. There is a need to guard against approaches which will deepen the often observed split between what students learn in the classroom and what they experience in the clinic. Teachers in college have a responsibility to try to bridge this gap through the use of teaching methods which include real clinical examples; 'the particular problems of patients'. So also do clinical teachers have a responsibility to encourage students to refer back to what has been found to be generally true, by having discussions about the knowledge base, by looking at the literature, at lecture notes, professional journals, etc.

In their study of supervisors of student teachers and health visitors Fish *et al.* (1991) found that there was very little attention to the knowledge base in the debriefing sessions with students. This shared responsibility for teachers of encouraging theory and practice to overlap, fosters what Jarvis (1983) describes as a 'community of learning'. These approaches guard against placing students in impossible situations where they find that they are unable to apply what they learnt in college, during their work experience.

Gaiptman and Anthony (1989), in discussing the development of self-directed learning in occupational therapy students, suggest that there is a conflict between the philosophies of the institutions running courses and those providing placements and running a service. The main aim of the institution being to expand and evaluate the body of knowledge, whereas the main aim of the placement agency is to provide a service to those who need it. This they say creates a dynamic tension, which can be productive, but can be difficult for students to reconcile. These ideas are explored further in the next chapter.

PRE-REGISTRATION COURSE DESIGN

A central aim of the curriculum in any sphere of professional education is to prepare the student to become a competent practitioner. Presumably curriculum developers believe that the overall design of the course and the syllabus content have a direct bearing on the preparation of students for the world of work. Those who have been involved in course design and development will be aware that although the main aim is straightforward the path to it is usually very complex. In health care courses, many different designs will be found; all include work experience which is supervised in some way. Various patterns of work experience can be found:

1. clinical practice taking place in college;
2. clinical practice arranged outside college but 'supervised' by a tutor appointed by college;
3. students going to a clinic outside college, supervised by practitioners;
4. students going to a clinic once or twice a week;
5. students going to a placement for a block of time as part of the term-time timetable.

In addition to these different patterns of work experience in the education programme, there are also variations in the way that placements are selected and monitored, or approved/accredited. In some fields the professional body takes the responsibility for approving the placement, while for other professions it is up to the individual course to select and monitor the placement. In some instances the pressure to find placements is such that there may be little choice.

A range of patterns is presumably fine because there are many and the courses are recognized, by the relevant professional and validating body, as being appropriate to get students to the starting line of competence on qualification. Nonetheless competence is unfortunately not an absolute, as we well know when we try to assess it. Therefore it is likely that some students enter their first job better prepared than others. Providing they are encouraged in their first post and maintain their motivation, they will grow to be practitioners who work to the maximum of their potential to provide a good quality service. It is inevitable that course designs vary, possibly the more they vary the richer will be the mix of practitioners entering the professional resource.

Those courses which have externally set and/or examined curricula will find that there are many frustrating restrictions with which they have to comply. What seems most important therefore is that college tutors and clinical teachers recognize the strengths and limitations of each individual course and thus ensure that measures are taken to balance up weak areas. For example, when students' main exposure to clinical work is in clinics on the site of the institution, do students also have the opportunity to work in the community and settings such as hospitals and schools, to identify and evaluate the differences. This is an area that has been addressed by a number of chiropody/podiatry degree programmes in the UK, which now include community placements in the students' work experience. Most fields have always included a range of placement experiences for students. Other issues to be addressed might be:

1. If students go into clinic mainly on a weekly basis do they also have the opportunity to see what it is like to be in clinic all the week?
2. Do students have the opportunity to work with cases on an intensive as well as an occasional basis?
3. If clinical experience is mainly patient-focused, does the curriculum also prepare them for the wider work context, such as the social and psychological factors which affect both clients and professionals?
4. Does the clinical practice attend only to the core of practice and not embrace the preparation of students to carry out administrative and managerial duties, as part of their work role? (see also Chapter 6).
5. Is the course design organized into tight subjet packages, which do not encourage students to integrate knowledge across subject boundaries?

There are some follow-up activities related to these issues at the end of the chapter.

These are some of the curriculum questions which need to be addressed, readers will be aware that there are many more. They are questions which need to be considered not only by course designers and college tutors, but also by clinical teachers, because all the aspects of the curriculum will have a marked effect on the learning experience of the student including the student as a learner within the 'clinical' setting.

A MODEL OF PROFESSIONAL PRACTICE

If we are to prepare students adequately for professional work then we need to consider what is involved in the practice of that profession. Professionals generally recognize three elements, these are:

- Knowledge
- Skills
- Attitudes

In 1983 I had the oportunity to try to develop an account of the work of the speech and language therapist by undertaking a detailed look at the work of four practitioners. The aim of the study was to reconsider the curriculum in the education of speech and language therapists, by starting at the reality of practice (Stengelhofen, 1984). The study of the speech and language therapists was undertaken through observations followed by in-depth interviews. The interviews in particular revealed the attitude of the therapists to their work. I was also interested to explore how knowledge gained during their pre-registration course was actually used in practice.

In considering the themes which emerged from the data in this study, the majority appeared to fit well into the elements of professional competence discussed by Jarvis (1983) (Box 1.3). It is not clear from this whether

Box 1.3 The elements of professional competence. Adapted from Jarvis (1983)

1. **Knowledge and understanding of:**	2. **Skills to:**	3. **Professional attitudes:**
Academic disciplines	Perform psychomotor procedures	Knowledge of professionalism
The psychomotor elements	Interact with others	Emotive commitment to professionalism
Interpersonal relationships		Willingness to perform professionally
Moral values		

Jarvis is presenting purely a list of headings, or whether he is actually presenting a model. It may therefore be useful to consider the three elements in more detail as well as to consider how the elements may relate to each other.

Knowledge

It was apparent from the observations and interviews that knowledge from subjects was not drawn on equally, nor was it used with equal levels of consciousness. Knowledge which is secure and well integrated appears to become embedded at a deep level and is used tacitly. One of the problems for clinical teachers is to make this deeply-embedded, tacit knowledge available to the learner, while new learning is applied consciously and is explicit. It can therefore be presumed that the knowledge of a new practitioner (or a student) is still held at the surface explicit level. The difficulty is to find out which parts are purely espoused (talked about) and which parts are actually used in solving the problems of practice.

In the data from the study there were two other themes which were of particular significance in relation to knowledge. These were knowledge awareness and experiential knowledge. It could be argued that new knowledge acquired through work experience will just go into the appropriate store of knowledge for a subject discipline. However, discussion with the clinicians showed that it did not fit clearly into a subject, that it was much more to do with how knowledge became used in their work with patients. In other words, that which was appropriate in the light of experience; how theories of a general nature related to the particular problems found in practice. Thus new knowledge was created specific to the individual practitioner's clinical needs. Presumably this creation of new knowledge also has to be within the student's experience, otherwise are they merely learning to become technicians?

It was also evident that the therapists reflected on their knowlede and the appropriateness of it to practice. If practitioners are going to be effective, experiential knowledge and knowledge awareness seem to be essential elements in a model of professional practice. This concept has been explored by Schon (1983) in his work *The Reflective Practitioner*. It is a concept which has importance in student learning, it will be taken up later in this book, and has been explored in the works' of Fish *et al.* (1989, 1991).

The data from the study suggested that the elements of professional competence interact strongly with each other and that a simple linear model as shown in Box 1.3, is inadequate. It is not clear why Jarvis includes 'Moral values' under 'Knowledge and understanding', although it can be argued that moral values must be based on the knowledge of such values. However they would seem to be far more influenced by and belonging to heading 3, 'Professional attitudes'.

In the same way, although there must be knowledge of interpersonal relationships, it appears under heading 2. Skills to:, 'interact with others'. No doubt the skill component of making relationships can be observed on the surface. However, unlike many other skills it is most strongly influenced by professional attitudes, and is therefore most meaningful under such a heading. Perhaps it should be part of a broader element entitled 'professional relationships'.

Techniques and procedures

The term skill, as used by Jarvis in the second heading, frequently has a narrow connotation. In the particular profession studied, and in the other professional groups we are concerned with, although a considerable amount of skill use can be observed, it would seem to be a term more appropriate to carrying out purely motor activities. Where the surface activity of a job is also informed by knowledge, based on problem identification the selection and design of appropriate procedures to change behaviour or a medical condition, the terms techniques and procedures would seem more appropriate.

The definition by Perrow (1965) is helpful:

Technology is a technique or a complex of techniques employed to alter materials (human and non-human, mental and physical) in an anticipated manner.

Perrow stresses that technology so defined, is informed by knowledge and would therefore not exclude reflection on the part of the practitioner. Like knowledge, techniques and procedures are presumably influenced by student learning and experience in practice. The role of continuing education is of particular importance in evaluating and updating techniques.

Attitudes

Heading 3, 'Professional attitudes' was evident in the data in the study. The handling of professional relationships formed a particularly important thread. This appeared to be most strongly influenced not by knowledge but by attitude, and therfore most properly belongs under the attitude heading. The data also gave evidence of the attitudes of the clinicians to their relationships with clients (patients), parents of clients and professional colleagues. There was only minimal evidence in the data of an awareness of the relationship with and influence of the employing authority.

Other themes in the data, planning and evaluation for example, seem to belong most appropriately under the attitude heading, because it is through the practitioner's attitude to work that motivation to plan and to evaluate is maintained. This is of central importance in relation to quality assurance.

It is evident therefore that although the elements and headings used by Jarvis are useful they do not encompass the relationships between the elements of professional practice, at least in the profession being examined in the study, and no doubt the same would apply in other health care professions. It is therefore necessary to put these headings into a conceptual framework, rather than leave them as a list of headings. Because the way we think about the work we do has a direct influence on the way this is relayed to the learners who are preparing to enter their chosen field.

A REVISED MODEL OF PRACTICE

A model is proposed which shows these elements at different levels. The surface of activities in health care are the techniques and procedures which can be observed, mainly when clinicians are working with clients/patients. It is within the interaction with these clients that various procedures can be undertaken. At the surface level there can also be observed the relationships with relatives, carers and other professionals.

Under the surface may be identified two deeper levels. At the first level, and perhaps the easiest to uncover through interviews with practitioners (or with students through questioning/tutorials, clinical debriefing sessions, etc.), is knowledge. However, knowledge needs to be divided into two levels, that is the surface explicit knowledge and the below-surface tacit level, described above. Below knowledge 'at a deeper level' are the attitudes to work, including the emotive commitment.

The revised model, as illustrated in Box 1.4, shows the three levels present in professional practice. The inclusion of feedback loops suggests that the practitioner considers and reflects on what is being done, evaluates this and if necessary, returns to the deeper levels to consider the alternatives.

Although the model generated was from practice in speech and language therapy it could be applied to all health care groups. The headings in Box 1.4 have been left blank so that the reader can fill in the details from the perspective of a particular professional sphere. The third follow-up activity, at the end of the chapter, suggests how you might approach this. This is a useful exercise for clinical teachers to undertake because all the elements have to be addressed in the curriculum. Furthermore, none of the elements can be left purely to college-based teaching or clinic-based teaching. Teachers in both situations need to be alert to the ways in which particular learning contexts and or methods can foster the development of the different elements of practice.

Box 1.4 A revised model of the elements of professional competence.
Adapted from Stengelhofen (1984)

Surface	1. TECHNIQUES AND PROCEDURES
	↑↓
1st Deep level	2. KNOWLEDGE AND UNDERSTANDING. AND KNOWLEDGE AWARENESS
	↑↓
2nd Deep level	3. ATTITUDES Giving meaning to what is done and influencing use of knowledge, techniques and procedures.
	↑
All levels influenced by:	Life experiences Pre-registration learning Work experience Continuing education Relationship with employing authority, work context e.g. hospital, school, clinic, private practice, etc.

THE MODEL OF PRACTICE AS IT RELATES TO HEALTH CARE COURSES

An examination of curricula in health care courses, from a range of institutions reveals that it is the first and second levels of the elements of competence which receive the main focus of attention. The way in which these two levels are handled rests on course designers and individual institution's views of the nature of, and the relationship between, theory and practice. If practice is seen largely as picking up skills through practice, then the first level of techniques and procedures will be viewed as particularly important. Sometimes techniques are viewed as the 'vocational' aspects and are assigned to a lower status, and the whole question of the relationship between theory and practice is evaded. With this approach, good but unthinking technicians will enter the field. In this context the insights referred to earlier by Argyris and Schon (1974) are helpful, because their concept of practice, which they term 'theories-of-action', incorporates the potential for a split. Over-attention, for example, to the skills/techniques may be at the expense of sound theory. Action is made up of espoused theories and theories in use. The acknowledgement of espoused theory, recognizes that practitioners, and especially students and beginners, can talk about what they ought to do. Use implies that a theory has been selected and brought into action in a particular instance. If this is accepted then it becomes important that:

1. Course content attends to theories relevant to practice.
2. Students are given ample opportunity to experience real practice during which they can learn to select from their knowledge store.
3. The course design encourages the student to move across discipline boundaries to consider all the possible solutions to problems encountered in practice.
4. Those teaching students in the work experience parts of the course need to be well prepared for the job.

COURSE DESIGNS TO MEET THE NEEDS OF LEARNERS ON HEALTH CARE COURSES

The majority of health care courses have followed well-tried, traditional approaches, or may even have been forced to adopt a 'rational' curriculum plan. This will be particularly true where courses are externally set and examined. The 'rational' approach is serialist and linear, biased to behavioural objectives and favouring step-by-step instruction. Assessment of students measures only the already predicted learning outcomes. There is therefore an assumption that it is comparatively easy to identify learning outcomes which are relevant to the reality of practice. Such an approach is almost bound to focus heavily on the first level of the model of practice (Techniques and procedures). It is therefore unlikely to consider all the factors relevant to the complexity of practice as well as to overlook the importance of choice in practice. It would seem that if health care work is not purely a matter of applying techniques then the pre-registration curriculum must adopt a course design which has greater flexibility than the 'rational' model allows.

Integrated course design

The model of practice proposed above, suggests that the practitioner needs access to knowledge from a range of subject disciplines. Course designers, therefore, should consider which curriculum models might encourage students to select from a range of knowledge. A study by Colditz and Sheehan (1982), on the impact of alternative methods of teaching in medical education, showed that subjects which were integrated did not encourage factual recall, but encouraged:

- Self educative skills
- Interpersonal skills
- Professional skills

We must therefore ask which of these qualities will be most important in the practitioner? Closely allied to this is the question of how the traditional balance is held between subject disciplines. Courses must include a number of disciplines to provide the knowledge base for practice: traditionally these have been clearly divided into subject areas.

Integration of subjects may be fought against by disciplines which see themselves as strong and influential, as integration involves the disturbance of existing authority structures both in interpersonal and hierarchical terms. The need for a particular discipline to become subordinate to the overall needs of a profession may be perceived as a threat and may therefore be opposed. This is an ongoing problem in the design and development of health care courses. Some fields have tackled this problem by undertaking all the teaching themselves. Although this solves the immediate problems of relevence and integration, it may foster a too narrow approach to the subject, not developing a proper theoretical base for further study. A certain richness will be lost which comes from lecturers from different fields contributing to the course. This not only enhances students' and therefore practitioners' lifelong learning potential, but facilitates joint teaching, clinical and research opportunities. It is also of importance in establishing the credibility of courses in the wider academic forum.

It can be argued that adoption of an integrated course in professional preparation encourages practitioners to use knowledge from across disciplines as well as to work more readily with other disciplines. Benor (1982) explored the value of integration in medical education in which 'each issue is illustrated from various points of view, the clincial problem being the tertiary level'. He stresses the value of integration in aiding the development of creative thinking, seen as central in medical practice and therefore essential in medical education. The same would apply in health care education. The development of creative thinking must be important in all health care fields, especially where interpersonal contacts are central and each client/patient presents unique needs.

Attitudinal development

The attitudinal level of competency is the most difficult to attend to in the curriculum. It is usually difficult to identify or even entirely missing from the course content. However the proposed model of practice suggests that it is this level which is the driving force for effective practice. Indeed it could be argued that as knowledge, techniques and procedures are subject to rapid change, while attitudes are slow to change, then it is the deepest attitudinal level that needs to be placed centrally in professional education. The curriculum therefore should include studies concerned with attitudes to professional practice. These should be introduced in the classroom but are probably most powerfully demonstrated in the work place. Attitudinal concepts needing exploration might be:

1. The need for continued learning throughout a career.
2. Awareness of strengths and limitations of a practitioner's knowledge.
3. Awareness that knowledge is quickly outdated.
4. Awareness of the value of team work.
5. The importance of interpersonal skills in effective practice.
6. How the institution affects the execution of practice.
7. Ethical issues related to practice, etc.
8. A holistic view of patients/clients.

Stressing the importance of the attitudinal level does not mean that it is not also essential that the syllabus is designed to equip the student with sound knowledge in a range of subjects to form the basis of present and future learning. However, if knowledge is projected as all-important there is a danger that, on entering practice, it will fossilize or drain away, unless it is found to be relevant to the needs of practice. Argyris and Schon stress the importance of the theory-of-action becoming individualized through opportunities for each student to be exposed to the reality of practice. Lack of knowledge in the new practitioner could therefore be explained by lack of opportunity for real work experience as a student. Other explanations might be:

1. Lack of relevance in the theories studied.
2. Lack of understanding by tutors of the possible relevance to problems of practice.
3. Lack of encouragement by clincial teachers to examine theory in trying to find solutions to clinical problems.
4. Hidden messages in the curriculum or from college tutors which suggest that certain subjects have a lower status. These are therefore not rigorously covered and thus perceived as irrelevant.

SUMMARY

College tutors and clinical teachers need to be aware of all the factors which are significant in course design and therefore influential in the way students learn to become competent practitioners. The clinical teacher just as much as the student is caught up in this network. The important factors can be summarized as follows.

1. Selecting a course design which is the most likely to foster the needs of students who will become health care professionals.
2. Ensuring that all the elements, knowledge, skills and attitudes are given attention in the curriculum.
3. Making explicit the areas of the curriculum related to professional development.
4. Establishing and maintaining links with the field of practice to avoid a split between college-based and clinic-based learning.
5. Re-examining the relevance of contributing disciplines.
6. Adopting a course design which does not denigrate the professional aspects of the course. Ensuring that the parts identified as 'practical' are given equal status to those parts identified as 'theoretical'.
7. Adopting a course design and using teaching methods which are most likely to:
   (a) foster a positive approach to working with patients;
   (b) aid creative thinking;
   (c) encourage problem solving;
   (d) encourage the selection of theories from the knowledge base;
   (e) foster the development of interpersonal skills.
8. Considering all the possible ways for students to experience the reality of work, in order for them to develop individual theories-in-use.
9. Consider how all teachers, including clinical teachers are prepared for and supported in their roles in the educational process.

FOLLOW-UP ACTIVITIES

1. List the choices you need to make in half a day at work.
2. Look again at the five questions about the organization of work experiences on p. 10. Consider each issue in relation to the course(s) attended by students you receive on placement. You may also want to add to the list of issues to be addressed by course designers.
3. Jot down aspects of your own work under the headings Knowledge, Skills and Attitudes. When you have considered these, complete your own model as shown in Box 1.4. Compare this with the complete model in Appendix A.
4. Take your treatment of one patient/client and make a list of the information/knowledge which you need to use in order to treat that patient/client effectively.
5. Think about the design of the course followed by the students who are placed in your clinic. What does the design of the course imply about the nature and status of practice? Do you consider that the course gives adequate opportunity for students to experience professional practice?.

6. Look at your professional journals – notice (and read!) articles related to clinical teaching.

REFERENCES

Argyris, C. and Schon, D. (1974) *Theory and Practice: Increasing Professional Effectiveness*, Jossey Bass, San Francisco.

Benor, D.E. (1982) Interdisciplinary integration in medical education: theory and method. *Medical Education*, **16**; no. 6, 355–61.

Bloom, B.S. (1954) *Taxonomy of Educational Objectives. Handbook I Cognitive domain*, D. McKay & Co, New York.

British Dietetics Association (1990) *Draft Model of Clinical Supervisors Education.* Unpublished paper, Health Care Professions Education Forum.

Colditz, G.A. and Sheehan, M. (1982) The Impact of Instructional Style on the Development of Professional Characteristics. *Medical Education*, **3**, no. 16, 127–32.

College of Occupational Therapists (1989) Adopting a Sequential Approach to Clinical Education.*British Journal of Occupational Therapy*, **52**, no. 1, 23–4.

Dickson, M. and Maxwell, M. (1985) The Interpersonal Dimension in Physiotherapy: Implications for Training. *Physiotherapy*, **71**, no. 1, 306–10.

Ellis, R. (1980) Social Skills Training for Interpersonal Professions, in Singleton, W., Spurgeon, P. and Stammers R. (eds) *The Analysis of Social Skills*, Plenum, New York.

Ellis, R. (ed.) (1988) *Professional Competence and Quality Assurance in the Caring Professions*, Chapman and Hall, London and New York.

Fish, D., Twinn, S. and Purr, B. (1989) *How to enable learning through professional practice*. West London Institute of Higher Education in association with Brunel University.

Fish, D., Twinn, S. and Purr, B. (1991) *Promoting Reflection: Improving Supervision of Practice in Health Visiting and Initial Teacher Training. How to enable Students to Learn Through Practice.* West London Institute of Higher Education in association with Brunel University.

Gaiptman, B. and Anthony, A. (1989) Contracting in Fieldwork Education: The Model of Self-directed Learning. *Canadian Journal of Occupational Therapy*, **56**; no. 1, 10–14.

Jarvis, P. (1983) *Professional Education*. Croom Helm, London.

Perrow, C. (1965) Hospitals: Technology, Structure and Goals, in March, J.G. (ed.) *Handbook of Organizations*, Rand McNally, Chicago.

Schwab, J.J. (1969) The Practical: A Language for the Curriculum. *School Review*, November, 1–23.

Schwab, J.J. (1971) The Practical: Arts of Eclectic. *School Review*, August, 493–541.

Schon, D. (1983) *The Reflective Practitioner: How professionals think in action*. Basic Books, New York.

Stengelhofen, J. (1984) *Curricula for Professional Education: an investigation into theory and practice in the work of speech therapists*. Unpublished MEd dissertation, University of Birmingham.

Stengelhofen, J.L (1990a) *Multidisciplinary Supervisors Course: Evaluation Report.* Unpublished paper, Yorkshire Health UK.

Stengelhofen, J. (1990b) *A Cross Professional Approach to Clinical Supervisors Courses.* Unpublished paper, Health Care Professions Education Forum.

Stengelhofen, J. (1991) Helping Students Learn in Clinical Settings. *Journal of the Association of Chiropody Teachers in the UK,* **6**, no. 1, 3–9.

2

Teaching and learning methods in the classroom and clinic

It is through developing the capability of students to learn effectively from their experiences that they will be able as professionals to be competent learners throughout their lives

Boud, D., 1985 (p. 68)

INTRODUCTION

Having looked broadly at curriculum design in the first chapter, teaching and learning methods will now be considered in the context of their appropriateness to different types of learning environment. Particular attention will be paid to those methods which can be adopted most easily in work experience, taking particular note of the demands on clinicians in being both a practitioner and a clinical teacher.

In the previous chapter some ideas about theory and practice in the pre-registration course, and how they related to curriculum design were considered. It is now necessary to look at the curriculum in more detail, especially those parts in which students undertake practical work. The clinical supervisor's/teacher's role cannot be seen within a vacuum; it relates to what has happened, is currently happening or what is going to happen to the student in the college-based parts of the course yet to come. It is easy to recognize that the teacher in the classroom has a major influence on student learning. From the memories of our own student experiences we will be aware of the marked influence which clinical teachers had on us. It was the clinical supervisors/teachers who were the main role models for our professional development and work.

TRADITIONAL TEACHING METHODS

Teaching and learning takes place both in the classroom and the 'clinic'. The term clinic is being adopted as a general term to cover all situations in which health professionals work. It might be, for example, a hospital department or ward, a community clinic a child development centre, a client's home or a school. Some approaches to teaching are much easier to carry out in the classroom setting and may be especially appropriate for certain kinds of learning. For example, when students in health care start to study physiology, the classroom may be an ideal setting to cover basic introductory information. However the laboratory would be a much more powerful context in which to grasp a real understanding of some physiological principles, through experimentation. There are, therefore, a number of possible ways and contexts in which learning may take place even within the college setting. The three main ways familiar to us all are:

- Lectures
- Seminars
- Tutorials

The lecture

The lecture is a common way of delivering information. It is the most cost-effective method, enabling the 'teaching' of a large number of students at one time. Students from different courses can be combined into the one lecture. Inevitably it becomes difficult for the lecturer to meet the specific syllabus needs of all students in the class. Those students who are later be required to apply the knowledge in a practical situation may find themselves in particular difficulties. Some health care students may have this kind of experience. Although the lecture is the most cost-effective method in staff:student ratio terms, it has been shown, unfortunately, not to be a very effective method in the promotion of student learning (Bligh, 1972).

Throughout the 1960s, '70s and '80s there has been clear evidence that the lecture method has many limitations in promoting student learning (Beard *et al.*, 1978; Bligh, 1972; Gibbs, 1982a; Habeshaw *et al*, 1982). Gibbs (1982b) outlines the unsound notions which are used to justify the use of lectures: lectures ensure that the ground is covered: lectures help students to learn factual material; lectures are inspirational; lectures ensure that students have a proper set of notes; students can pay attention for up to 50 or 60 minutes. He stresses that these are all false claims.

There are also views held that if students do not have to attend lectures they do not do any work. It has been a problem for some health courses to reduce both the amount of contact time for students and to make more use of a range of teaching methods. With the development of degree programmes in all fields and the associated and consequent development of research, there is likely to be more rapid change in the knowledge base. Gibbs (1982b) points out that alongside this are changes in communications technology, so that it has become easier to find things out. Consequently 'the need to know becomes less crucial and the ability to find out becomes paramount'.

Some students like lectures as a method because little demand is placed on the individual at the time. Students who are used to a large amount of lectures, from previous educational experience, may resist a change to other forms of teaching. The lecture can, in fact, form a useful introduction to a subject and provide an 'advance organizer'/cognitive map or framework (Ausubel, 1968), in which to receive and organize other knowledge.

Where courses have an externally set and assessed curriculum, there may be a tendency to make heavy use of the lecture method. This is because it is the only way that those responsible for running the course gain some, albeit false, re-assurance from knowing that the syllabus has at least been covered. This cover may only go as far as the topic appearing on a lecture programme list. Some health care courses tend to have a very high staff–student contact ratio, especially in the form of lectures. This suggests that there is an overloading of the factual content which may actually prevent students from developing a deep approach to learning (Entwistle, 1981). It is therefore necessary to question whether or not students are helped to become self-directed, self-motivated learners through this high degree of contact.

Although the lecture can be a good method for introducing students to new material, and to provide a framework of knowledge to be expanded through private study, students frequently believe that all the information they need is contained in the lecture. Gibbs and Harland (1987) suggest that staff in educational institutions should consider the question, 'Given the nature of our subject, including the constraints of validation and staff:student ratios, are there different ways of teaching or different emphasis, that would allow its aims and objectives to be more successfully achieved.'

Entwistle and Hounsell (1977) stress the importance of matching the teaching methods with the best way of achieving the learning objectives. The slot termed 'lecture' is greatly enhanced if other teaching methods are incorporated, such as buzz groups, snowballing and brainstorming (Beard, 1970). In these methods the whole group is broken down into small groups, to encourage individual thinking and participation. In **buzz groups** students are asked to work in small groups (4 or 5 students) to solve a problem, or discuss some controversial issue. A spokesperson for the group is appointed to report back to the class. The lecturer usually draws the main points together. In **snowballing** each student is asked first of all to write down his/her own ideas/thoughts, then to share these with a neighbour. When this has been done the newly formed pair share and compare their ideas with another pair. The group of four may then discuss with another group of four, and so it goes on, the snowball gradually getting bigger, until everyone has been included, or the discussion halted at any point. In **brainstorming** individual students are asked to write down as many ideas as they can, on a certain topic. They should be encouraged to write everything that comes into their head on the topic, however ridiculous it may seem initially. After a given time the ideas generated by individuals are discussed in small groups, to sift, consider and summarize them. French (1989) gives a useful account of using small group teaching methods with physiotherapy students. She makes the important point that these methods can also be used in the teaching of patients.

The seminar

Seminars take place in a group smaller than the whole class. The ideal number is considered to be seven or eight. As a method the seminar should be more *student-* than staff-centred. The degree of student-centredness will depend on the approach of the tutor. There may be exploration of a topic already introduced in lectures, or there may be consideration of a new topic which students have prepared for by recommended reading. Although the seminar is mainly concerned with the cognitive aspects of learning, that is:

- Ideas
- Concepts
- Principles,

seminars can also provide an opportunity to explore feelings and attitudes. Seminar topics to explore attitudes might be: elderly people, children with special needs going into mainstream schools, bereavement, ethnic differences, etc. Seminar methods could also be used in a clinical setting; this could be most easily set up where a number of students attend at the same time. Hospital-based student nurses are the most likely to have the opportunity to work with a small group. Chiropody, orthoptics and physiotherapy students may attend clinics in small groups. It is worth remembering that students can do very well on their own in small group discussions, sometimes they do just as well as with a teacher there!

The tutorial

The tutorial should place even more emphasis on the work of the individual student, their progress and their learning needs. The tutorial may focus on the preparation or review of an individual piece of work. Projects and dissertations require a good deal of individual tutorial time. Tutorials are also appropriate for consideration of case reports or case studies. In essence, clinical teachers are using tutorial methods with individual students when discussing progress with clinical work. In this instance the learning opportunity not only explores the knowledge base, but also covers the application of this knowledge to problems in patients, as well as, it is hoped, considering the student's feelings and attitudes.

The clinic-based tutorial provides an excellent opportunity for helping the student to explore feelings and attitudes generated whilst actually working with patients. College-based tutorials can form an important link between college and clinic-based learning. Care should be taken that such tutorials do not provide a forum for complaint or implied criticism of what may be a decision made by a clinician. In line with the earlier definition of theory and practice it is best for the classroom teacher to focus on general principles as a basis for discussion, with students mentally referring across to particular patient examples. In a clinical tutorial, the case of a particular patient would be taken as the starting point for the discussion, to refer across to what is found to be generally true in the knowledge base.

TEACHING METHODS WHICH FOSTER APPLICATION

Laboratory work

Some college-based teaching methods may naturally have a much more practical focus. For the science student, work carried out in a laboratory is an obvious example. 'Laboratory teaching' is included in health care courses and may be used in a number of subjects, for example in the teaching of anatomy and physiology, behavioural sciences and computer skills for all health students, audiology for speech and language therapy students, optics for orthoptics students, etc. Indeed, the clinic might also be regarded as the laboratory for the health student. Perhaps if viewed in this way, clinical experience would be given a higher status as an essential facility, rather than as an optional extra, which it is seen as by some institutions. Unlike most laboratory situations the material to be used is human, this makes the provision more complex to set up, as well as making the learning task more difficult and less controllable for the students. An institution might regard a college-based clinic as the laboratory for the health student, rather than those clinics which students attend away from college.

Workshop activities

The definition of a 'workshop' is never an easy one: is it a place or an activity? Possibly it is both. Workshop usually refers to a range of practically-based activities, which should be undertaken by students in a prescribed period.

It may also refer to a place where students can go and work on their own, particularly on the practical aspects of their studies. Some examples might be: orthotics workshops for splint making in chiropody and occupational therapy; carrying out a detailed speech and language analysis from taped data, in speech and language therapy; practising the Cover test and ocular testing in orthoptics, etc. Interactive videos could be used to develop communication and counselling skills.

The difficulty of 'experimenting' with patients makes it imperative that, in college, a range of teaching and learning methods is used that prepare students, as far as possible, for patient contact. Although these may be classroom-based they are specifically designed to bridge the clinic–classroom gap.

Role play

Role play exercises can be used in college as a valuable way of preparing students to carry out certain elements of professional practice. It can include students playing themselves as well as playing the role of others. Staff may also participate. Role play may be particularly useful in developing the following:

- Interactive skills
- Interviewing skills
- Counselling skills
- Case history taking
- Working in groups

The use of role play in helping to develop management skills is discussed in Chapter 6.

Situations are carefully set up with a scenario clearly described, with rules assigned to the individual's involved. Examples of role play scenarios can be seen Boxes 2.1 (a) and (b). It may be useful for scenes to be replayed with the student taking on different roles; this can deepen the understanding of the situation and the experiences of all the people involved. In health work, concepts such as the categorization of patients, and the clinician's role and status can be explored. Role play also helps students to consider people as a whole and not as diagnostic entities, such as 'stroke patients', 'Parkinson patients', 'diabetics', or 'Collis fractures'; such terminology ignores the centrality and value of the individaul in favour of that of the condition. Role play is a very helpful bridging activity as it allows students to move nearer to the experiences of which they may be fearful, and to make mistakes which will not have any serious consequences.

For the potential of role play to be fully explored it should be audio- or video-recorded. Video-recording is the more valuable, especially when patient–student communication is being considered, as it will also capture the

Box 2.1(a) Characters in a role play scenario. Adapted from Rachel David, Birmingham Polytechnic, BSc Speech and Language Pathology and Therapeutics

---

In the role play students work in pairs or threes, according to the characters in the scenario. Each is assigned to a character. Students do not know what information the other characters have been given. Another student may be involved as an observer/reporter.

SCENARIO ONE

Information to student A. You are Mrs H. a patient on a medical ward, you suffered a stroke last week. You are unable to stand and you have lost the use of your right hand. Your talking has been affected and you can speak only in single words. It is 7.45 p.m. and you are sitting in the chair beside your bed. Your husband promised to come to see you at 7 p.m. sharp this evening and he is always punctual. Your daughter is staying at your home and she is expecting a baby next month. You are worried because your husband hasn't arrived, and you think it may be because your daughter has gone into labour. You want to ask the nurse to 'phone your home to find out what has happened.

Information to student B: Nurse. You are the staff nurse on a very busy medical ward. Mrs H. is a middle aged woman who had a stroke last week. She is unable to stand and walk or to use her right hand. She also has some difficulty talking. Visiting time is at 7 p.m. As you pass Mrs H's bed at 7.45 p.m. you notice that she is sitting in her chair and that she does not have any visitors. You know that her husband cannot always manage to visit in the evenings. You are anxious to get the patients ready for bed so that you will be ready to hand over to the night nurse at 9 p.m. You ask Mrs H., as she has no visitors, if she would like you to help her get ready for bed.

SCENARIO TWO

Information to student A: You are an elderly lady Mrs S. who lives alone and you had a stroke 2 months ago. You are now in a geriatric hospital. It has taken a long time to get over your initial confusion but you are now aware of where you are and how long you have been in the hospital. However, you are still having a lot of difficulty in talking in sentences. Your daughter is coming to visit you and you are very anxious to know:

1. Whether anyone is taking care of your cat.
2. What is happening to your pension?

Information to student B: You are Mrs S's daughter. She is an elderly lady who lives on her own. She has been in a geriatric hospital for 2 months

Box 2.1(a) (continued)

following a stroke. You live in three-bedroomed house with your husband
two young children. You have a full-time job as a school secretary, which
you enjoy very much. You have been coming to visit your mother regularly
since she has been in hospital, but she has only seemed to recognize you
in the last 2 or 3 weeks. You still cannot follow much of what she says.
You have just seen her doctor, who says that she will never be able to
live on her own again. You want to talk to her about what the doctor has
said and about the arrangements for when she is ready to leave hospital.

Box 2.1(b) Format for role play scenarios. Adapted from Rachel David,
Birmingham Polytechnic, BSc Speech and Language Pathology and Therapeutics

Students are given five minutes to act out the situation. Following the role
play, discussions cover;
  what problems the individuals had encountered, in their adopted roles;
  what they had felt in the situation, and if they were surprised about
    the way that they felt;
  the ways in which the individual's agenda can influence the giving and
    receiving of information;
  how else the role might have been played, and how this would have
    influenced the development of the role play;
  what each of the student's learnt out of the role play experience.

non-verbal expression, e.g. eye contact, facial expression, gesture and posture.
The student can then replay the video, and practise different styles, having
first observed how he/she came over. Initially, students will find role play
and video-recording anxiety provoking, and nervousness may well inhibit their
natural responses. It is important, therefore, for them to have several
opportunities for role play and watching themselves on video, so that they
get used to it and then behave more naturally. It is advantageous to introduce
students to audio- and video-recording early on in their course, so that they
become used to the experience prior to its use to aid learning in clinical settings.

Another advantage of working with a group of students is that they can
more easily constitute a group for role play. It is a teaching method that could
also fruitfully be used across disciplines. If students from different fields are
used it prevents the players getting too caught up in the content of the clinical
field and therefore helps the participants to focus on the process. There are
ideas on the use of role play in Hawkings and Shohet (1989), which have

special application for those professions working primarily through the interpersonal medium.

In dietetics, clinical psychology and speech and language therapy, where the focus is generally on verbal exchange, audio-recording should be used if video-recording is not available. Recording encourages objective feedback and enables student and teacher to focus on specific behaviours during the subsequent analysis of the role play session (see also Chapter 7). Areas of strength can be explored as well as those which present difficulties and need modification. Observation skills are improved. Opportunity for the exploration of feelings should be provided. Furthermore, students can can also be given the message that qualified clinicians have to analyse their own behaviour.

Patient simulation exercises

Patient simulation exercises are a way of getting even nearer to the clinical reality. In these exercises, actors are trained to play specific cases. This allows the student to begin to feel what it may be like to have interface with real clients/patients, but at the same time to feel safe and be able to explore thoughts and motivations which guide their decisions and actions. In this kind of exercise video- and audio-recording is essential, allowing for analysis after the session.

If actors are not available, then staff or peers can be used in the same way. A lecturer may be excellent at playing the physical and psychological characteristics of a patient with a specified disorder. This method may also be found to be effective in the clinical setting. It can be used, for example, for practising the physical handling of patients, or practising the managing of difficulties encountered by the student in relating to particular patients. The student can 'replay' the clinical experience using either a peer or a clinician. This approach may help the student to achieve more insight into what went on in the session. This understanding may be enhanced by the student playing the patient and someone else playing the student, in a way in which they think the student behaved, thus enabling the student to feel what it is like to be on the other side. Ideas for simulation exercises can be found in Watts (1990).

Audio and video-recorded material

Use should be made of recorded material in the classroom. Recordings may be professionally prepared to support classroom teaching. Lecturers who carry out clinical work have the advantage of being able to illustrate lectures with recorded cases known to them. Well-prepared recordings, if accompanied by handouts can provide excellent opportunities for independent learning. They will be invaluable for illustrating the nature and management of cases which students may not have much opportunity to meet in their clinical placements.

Recorded material may provide students with their first experience of patient observation of a certain condition. In some instances students' observations and understanding may be deepened by enlargement and 'freezing' of a structure to be examined, by replaying on video, or film. For example, in orthoptics an enlarged picture of eye movement, can be replayed and each frame examined to develop diagnostic skills. In speech and language therapy, video-recording of patterns of feeding and swallowing, or palatal movement in speech, obtained through nasendoscopic examination can be replayed many times. Examples may also be provided to introduce students to the physical and psychological handling of patients. Clinical situtations where an observer may not be easily accommodated, such as counselling and sometimes history taking (in initial interviews) may be introduced through recordings, with the permission of the patients concerned. Material may also be used which is far from ideal, encouraging students to spot the 'deliberate mistakes' and thus begin to identify good practice.

Learning partnerships

In the college environment the student has ready-made opportunities for working collaboratively with other students. There is good evidence that students can progress through working with each other, even with no tutor present (Goldschmid, 1988). Students undertaking distance-learning courses, such as those run by the Open University in the United Kingdom, often form themselves into self-help groups.

Students who are together in clinic have a potential advantage as they have the opportunity to receive mutual support, share experiences, ask each other questions which they may feel inhibited in asking staff, plan together, role play together, and observe each other undertaking clinical work and discussing it afterwards. Clinical teachers who work with more than one student should consider if they have fully explored the ways the students could support each other in their learning. The second follow-up activity at the end of the chapter suggests that you do this.

CLINIC-RELATED EXPERIENCES

Many teaching methods based in or organized from college attempt to introduce students to the real work experience. For example, opportunities may be arranged for students to observe and/or work in a variety of settings or to undertake activities which introduce them to experiences which are related to, but not the same as, the professional target. For example, working in a home for the elderly, or in a school (Box 2.2). Although these may be arranged by the course prior to the clinical practice, there may be occasions where

Box 2.2 Experiences related to students' future work in clinical settings

1. Working on a ward alongside nurses in order to understand the role of the nurse and to try to understand the hospital experience from the patient's perspective.
2. Working in an old peoples' home or day centre, for those professional groups who undertake work with the elderly.
3. Visits with other health staff, for example health visitors, for those students who study child development, in preparation for working with children.
4. Attendance for periods of time to playgroups, schools, etc. for those whose work involves a lot of contact with children.
5. Visits to other departments to observe patients who require multiprofessional services. This helps to take the pressure off the student as the 'up-front' professional, and helps them to achieve a more holistic view of a patient's needs. Students should be well prepared in observation skills, before undertaking such visits.

it would be legitimate for the clinical teacher to build similar experiences into the placement programme. For example, visiting patients in their homes (if this is not routinely done in the clinical field) in order to help the student gain a more realistic view of the patient's needs and problems, without having to take on the specific professional role. Students studying 'remedial' work with pre-school children could interact with children in a nursery or playgroup setting, if they do not already have experience of being with young children. Such arrangements may not be viewed as legitimate, in what is identified as clinical time however it may be the only way forward for a student who is having difficulty with coping at a basic level.

Nevertheless the most valuable way of learning about the job is actually to do it. The student must have had suitable preparation and, during work experience, had time to **analyse, reflect** and **plan**. Boud (1985) suggests that in experiential learning the student needs to recapture as much as possible of what has happened by

- Returning to the experience
- Attending to feelings
- Re-evaluating the experiences

Some clinicians may argue that for a student to work with a reduced case-load is not introducing them to the reality of work. But, manual dexterity and other skills can only be built up from a slow start. Carrying out complex clinical procedures requires time to check that all elements have been carried out correctly. Diagnosing a condition and planning the next step requires constant consideration and re-consideration of the information available and cannot be processed at speed by the learner. It is worth remembering that when we first learn to do anything we cannot use all the required skills and thought processes concurrently, nor can we perform the new skills at maximum speed. We do not learn to be competent drivers by driving down the fast lane of a motorway. It is obviously wise for students gradually to increase their case-load as they move towards qualification.

THE LEARNING ENVIRONMENT OF THE CLINIC

In spite of the possible overlaps of teaching methods for the classroom and the clinic, it is fully recognized that the clinic is a radically different learning environment from the college-based classroom. A number of factors affect the clinic as a learning environment, some of which are suggested below. They appear to fall into three main groups: those related to the environment, those which are problems for the student and those which are problems for the clinical teacher:

Problems created by the clinical environment

1. Although the clinic is potentially very active it can be passive for the student, especially at an early observational stage, if the student's role is not clearly defined and their observations are not organized and focused. Helping students to be effective observers will be considered in Chapter 5.
2. Some of the best learning opportunities are those which are unscheduled, and may therefore not be fully explored.
3. Plans may often be disrupted because of a change in a patient's condition, the late arrival of transport, etc.
4. Teaching in clinic often occurs in an open situation, subject to scrutiny by the public and colleagues. This brings added pressures on both teachers and learners.

Problems for the student

1. The student may not have long to settle down into the clinical setting. This can be particularly difficult if the student had a timetable where the week is a mix of clinic and college attendance.
2. The student is very often removed from peer group support.
3. If students are unsure of their role in the work setting they may behave in uncharacteristic ways; for example, they need to know when they should or should not help or participate.

4. Students are subject to a high level of anxiety, which affects their learning. If this is not recognized by the clinical teacher the anxiety-provoked behaviours may be misconstrued.
5. What is visible on the surface of the clinical practice often appears simple. There is, therefore, a danger that the observing student will think that carrying out the treatment is simple. Furthermore, unless helped, students will not be aware of the thought processes underlying the clinical decisions, *preceding* the actions or the thinking going on *during* the 'handling' of a patient.

Problems for the clinical teacher

1. In the classroom the teacher can exercise a considerable amount of control, in contrast to the clinic where the teaching is related, but secondary, to patient care. As the patient will very often be present, there is far more risk involved. This element of risk may produce considerable anxiety both in the student and the clinical teacher, as well as in the patient, of course (Munroe, 1988).
2   The clinician's main role and first responsibility is treating patients, unlike the classroom teacher whose first responsibility is teaching students.
3. The clinical teacher has to respond to the needs of patients, other staff, parents, spouses and carers of patients, transport and administration, etc.
4   The clinician may not have had any preparation for the clinical teaching role and may feel considerably ill at ease within it.
5   The clinician needs to help the student to be aware of the knowledge base to be drawn on in the treatment of patients. Real problems are often complex and the student will need help in making sense of them, and help in relating them back to what may have been covered in the classroom. The earlier discussion on the relationship between theory and practice is of great importance here. A small clinical resource, including textbooks, copies of journals and single articles should be made available for student use. When clinical teachers photocopy and share articles, students may reciprocate. The student's self-esteem will be greatly enhanced if they feel they can share their own newly acquired knowledge with the clinical teacher.
6. Experienced clinicians are often unaware of the knowledge base which prompts their actions; the student may therefore act as a catalyst in helping to unearth concepts embedded over time. Working with a student is a great time for reviewing the appropriateness of clinical thinking in the context of current knowledge.
7. Pressure on clinicians may lead them to be over-directive, which discourages self-motivated, self-directed learning in the student.

8. What is *done* by the clinician is probably more powerful than what is said, and is probably even more powerful than what is said by the teacher in the classroom. It is very difficult to control the hidden agenda. The above points about the clinic as a learning environment need to be considered further in the context of your own field.

BRIDGING THE CLINIC–CLASSROOM GAP

The student stands on the bridge between the clinic and the classroom. Both situations present a number of learning opportunities. It is hoped that what is explored in the classroom and what is experienced in the clinic will, for the most part, tie up, but this does not always happen. Alternatives and different procedures are not bad things, especially if the student has been prepared for the differences and is later encouraged to explore and evaluate them, either in clinic or through debriefing sessions in college and through further study.

Teachers, in whatever context, have a responsibility to try to help learners keep in view and bring together what has happened at both ends of the bridge. It is worth considering how the potential gap between the classroom and the clinic can be avoided. It is particularly important that the student views the clinic as a learning environment just as much as the classroom. Making the student feel welcome in a clinic, is a prerequisite in creating an atmosphere conducive to learning. How little we remember when we feel anxious. Teachers in a classroom do not always achieve a conducive environment. Accommodation needs to be found in the working environment where the student and clinical teacher can discuss progress in private. Seating arrangements should, if possible, not be too formal.

Just as in the classroom, it is important to set out for the student the framework for a session, for example: 'This morning we're going to see four patients, some on the ward and some in outpatients, who all have (condition X), I believe that you've had some lectures in college on this?..
That's fine. I want you to observe their treatment, but also to help me with them, perhaps if they need to be brought from the waiting area or they need to transfer from bed to chair. I'll tell you at the time how I want you to help. Next week I want you to treat one of the patients, perhaps you'd like to decide who you'd like to work with. At the end of the morning we'll talk about each patient and I'll want you to try to describe how the condition presents in each of them. How do you feel about this? ....
You could spend the next ten minutes deciding what you need to remember to look at'. This setting of the agenda before the session and the learning experience in it, facilitates the learning; putting the student at ease in

Box 2.3 Bridging the clinic–classroom gap

In the classroom	In the clinic
Use of video of real patients referring forward to the clinical experience.	Provide patient examples for topics covered in the classroom.
Demonstrations teacher/student, students practice on each other.	Demonstration on student, use clinical teacher or other student as a model.
Introduce the student to a number of different 'schools of thought' so they are able to select the most appropriate in a particular patient-related instance.	Perhaps one approach isn't working; encourage student to look back in notes etc to (i) identify possible alternatives and (ii) explore along with clinical teacher those that might be relevant to the patient concerned. Point out relevant/recent articles in professional publications – read, discuss, try out if appropriate.
Introduce the student to a number of different ways of carrying out a specific procedure.	Ask students about the way they have been taught in college; make clear that although you may have a preferred way, you acknowledge that there are others. Allow the student to try out alternatives.
Use problem-solving activities to foster a problem-solving approach to clinical work.	Don't tell the student too much; try not to be over-directive; let students come up with ideas on their own. Encourage the student to question; yes this can be frightening!
Encourage students to be self-directed learners from the beginning of the course.	Allow students to take responsibility for what they decide to do, and what they do with specific patients. Allow them to learn from own mistakes. Let them see your mistakes too; explore these as a learning opportunity.

Box 2.3 (continued)

Do not criticize the knowledge and work undertaken by clinicians. This may happen inadvertently.	Do not criticize the knowledge and work undertaken by college tutors, or denigrate their motives for having a lecturing job.
Provide clinically-oriented resources: examples of treatment materials; audio- and video-recordings of patients, different conditions and their treatment. Students should have easy access to these.	Provide a small library which includes journals, copies of journal articles. Encourage students to use postgraduate library facilities.

Run joint seminars
Undertake collaborative research
Participate in clinical teaching courses together

knowing what they will be required to do, as well as alerting the student cognitively to the area of knowledge to be considered ('advance organiser'; Ausubel, 1968).

Later in the day the student and clinical teacher discuss the condition and the treatment of the four patients. At the end of the discussion: 'You made some good observations of the patients. Perhaps you need to be a bit more careful to notice _____ How do you think you'll remember? Yes, it would be a good idea to look over your lecture notes on the assessment, before next time. Do you know if there are any videos in college? I'm pleased that you've chosen Mr. A.; you'll need his notes. You'll need to think about the aims and objectives for his treatment and think about the methods and what you'll need. We could check over your plans first thing tomorrow'.

It is clear that this clinician has in mind the total learning experience, clinic and classroom for the student, and is sure to bridge the gap between them. There are many approaches which can be used by college tutors and clinical teachers, which help to bring the learning experiences together. Some other ideas are suggested in Box 2.3.

Many other ideas for bridging the gap will evolve if classroom teachers and clinical teachers have opportunities to meet, and not only in the context of student progress. Perhaps the most valuable approach is the chance to understand each other's working stituation; Benson and Martin (1987) describe the exchange of jobs between a lecturer and a clinician, in occupational therapy.

Both showed similar anxieties and apprehension to those experienced by students. The lecturer was particularly anxious on going to clinic. So how much more anxious must students be? One finding from the experiment was that students had not viewed the lecturer as a 'proper occupational therapist'. Both participants recommended similar exchanges would be valuable to other staff.

FOLLOW-UP ACTIVITIES

1. Consider the points on pages 33–35 on the clinic as a learning environment. Evaluate how each point is relevant to: (a) your own field, (b) you as a clinical teacher and (c) the particular context in which you work. Extend the list from the teaching experiences you have had in your work with students.
2. If you have two or more students to teach at one time in your clinical setting, review the opportunities they have for using partnership in learning.
3. Look again at Box 2.2, then list any opportunities you think could be of value in your own field, which you or the course could arrange. Discuss your ideas with the course leader.
4. Look at the clinical programme for the student(s) you are working with, identify where the times are for reflecting on what has gone on. Discuss this with the student(s) concerned. In the light of your discussions build into the programme more 'thinking space'.
5. Find out if a job swop has ever been considered in your field – would it be possible; would you be interested?
6. Look again at Box 2.3, consider the suggestions in column 2. Are they appropriate for your work? Evaluate your own use of each idea.

REFERENCES

Ausubel, D.P. (1968) *Educational Psychology: A Cognitive View*, Holt Reinhart and Winston, New York.

Boud, D. (1985) How to help students learn from experience, in Cox. K.R. and Ewan, C.E. (eds) *The Medical Teacher*, 2nd edn., Churchill Livingstone, Edinburgh.

Beard, R.M. (1970) *Teaching and Learning in Higher Education*, Penguin Education, Harmondsworth, UK.

Beard, R.M., Blight, D.A. and Harding, A.G. (1978) *Research into Teaching Methods in Higher Education*, 4th edn., S.R.H.E., Guildford.

Benson, S. and Martin, J. (1987) A Liverpool Tale. *British Journal of Occupational Therapy*, **50**, no. 11, 381–3.

Bligh, D. (1972) *What's the Use of Lectures?* Penguin Education, Harmondsworth, UK.

Entwistle, N. (1981) *Styles of Learning and Teaching*, John Wiley, New York.

Entwistle, N. and Hounsell, D. (1977) *How Students Learn: Implications for Teaching and Learning in Higher Education*. Institute for Research and Development in Post Compulsory Education, University of Lancaster.

French, S. (1989) Student Centred Learning. *Physiotherapy*, **75**, no. 11, 678–80.

Gibbs, G.P. (1982a) *Twenty Terrible Reasons for Lecturing*, Occasional Paper, Standing conference for Educational Development Services in Polytechnics.

Gibbs, G.P. (1982b) *Better Teaching or Better Learning*, in Habeshaw, T., Fothergill, R., Gibbs G.P. and Heron, J. (eds) *Three Ways to Learn*, Occasional Paper 12, Bristol Polytechnic. Standing conference for Educational Development Services in Polytechnics.

Gibbs, G.P. and Harland, J. (1987) Approaches to Teaching in Higher Education. *British Educational Research Journal*, **13**, 159–73.

Goldschmid, M. (1988) Parrianage: Students Helping Each Other, in Boud, D. (ed.) *Developing Student Autonomy in Learning*, Kogan Page, London.

Habeshaw, T., Fothergill, R., Gibbs, G.P. and Heron, J. (1982) *Three Ways to Learn*, Occasional Paper 12, Bristol Polytechnic, Standing conference for Educational Development Services in Polytechnics.

Hawkins, P. and Shohet, R. (1989) *Supervision in the Helping Professions*, Open University Press, Buckingham, UK.

Munroe, H. (1988) Modes of Operation in Clinical Supervision: How Clinical Supervisors Perceive themselves. *British Journal of Occupational Therapy*, **51**, no. 10, 338–43.

Watts,N. (1990) *Handbook of Clinical Teaching*, Churchill Livingstone, Edinburgh.

3

The special job of teaching
students in clinic

INTRODUCTION

This chapter opens with a discussion about those staff who are involved in teaching and monitoring students in the practical parts of their pre-registration course. Consideration is given to the particular needs of adult learners. There is a section on styles of teaching and learning and how these may affect the relationship between the teacher and the learner. The chapter ends with a consideration of a number of other factors which may affect teaching and learning in clinical settings; there is particular emphasis on interpersonal communication between the student and clinical teacher.

NAMES AND ROLES

In the first chapter the different terms in use were noted, such as: clinical educator, clinical instructor, clinical teacher, clinical trainer, clinical tutor, field work teacher/instructor/tutor, practical teacher, and clinical supervisor. In this book the term **clinical teacher** is adopted because the author considers that it best describes the job to be done. It indicates an active role for both clinician and student. These concepts of teaching and learning are different from those which have previously been dominant in the apprentice-type model. In the latter, the emphasis is on the student observing and doing, having modelled the doing on the clinician's behaviour.

Although this book is devoted mainly to the teaching of students in clinical settings, it is recognized that clinicians also have a teaching role with patients. Many of the principles explored will be applicable to the teaching of both students and patients. For the new clinical teacher this job of teaching patients/clients is a useful starting point, as it can be used to explore some of the generic skills posessed by all clinicians which can be transferred from the job of working with patients to working with students. Relevant skills which can be transferred are:

- observational
- interactional
- counselling
- passing on knowledge
- instructional

Marson (1990), in discussing ward teaching in nursing, suggests that the qualities needed for being a good teacher are similar to those of being a good nurse: empathy, sensitivity and an ability to listen and respond appropriately. The parallels between being a clinician (or nurse) and being a clinical teacher are generally positive, although there is sometimes a danger of the clinician becoming too much of a therapist ('quasi-therapist') to the student, whether because they are drawn into this by the student or they feel that this should be part of the role (Hawkins and Shohet, 1989). This may be more of a trap for those professionals who carry out their job primarily through the inter-personal medium and therefore make frequent and legitimate use of counselling in their work with patients. Being a 'therapist' for the student may not be the best way to help them. If skilled counselling is needed this should probably come from another source. Clinical teachers need to preserve their very specialized clinical skills for working with patients and not be drained by counselling students. The clinical teacher (and nurse tutor) is exposed to considerable emotional pressure in having to deal concurrently with the physical, psychological and social needs of patients. Too much involvement with the emotional needs of students will add to the emotional pressure on clinicians. Where particular counselling support is needed, advice should be sought from the institution which has placed the student. Institutions make counselling provision for both the academic and personal needs of students, these resources should be referred to where students are in difficulties. It is important that clinical teachers are fully aware of the support systems available for students.

A number of different personnel may be involved with the clinical teaching of students. In some professions classroom teachers/college lecturers, although appointed as lecturers to an institution may also teach students in the clinical environment, either in an on-site clinic or in a community or hospital setting. In some professions, e.g. nursing and physiotherapy, a clinical tutor may be appointed by the institution, but the majority, or all, the teaching will be done in clinical settings. The covert expectation here is that clinical tutors are master clinicians who know *everything* about the field, placing them in an inherently stressful role. This type of appointment may also imply that college lecturers are not capable of doing competent clinical work and that clinicians are not capable of teaching, in the sense of delivering a lecture. Furthermore, and possibly more seriously, it may imply that the clinical tutor is not capable of teaching in the classroom and therefore that teaching and learning in the clinic is of a lower status than teaching and learning in the classroom. Therefore, what is seen as practice (clinical) is of lower status than that which is seen as theoretical (classroom).

The role of the clinical teacher may be envisaged in a number of different ways according to the profession and the institution. What is important is that both the course team and the clinicians are aware of, and make explicit, what the role is. This should be done through course documentation, clinical handbooks, etc., but will also be picked up from the hidden agenda in the course design and the behaviour of lecturers towards clinical teachers. Full discussion of the role needs to take place in the interface between those responsible for managing and teaching the course in the classroom, and the clinical teachers.

The importance of the relationship between the clinical teachers and the institution running the course is clearly of great importance. There are, however, several other important interfaces related to running a course, which may affect teachers, in both clinical and classroom settings. Some of these are shown in Box 3.1.

Box 3.1 Important interfaces in running a course. Stengelhofen (1991)

The course	The professional body
The course	The validating body
The course	The institution
The clinical teachers	The course
The clinical teachers	The lecturers
The clinical teachers	The employers
The students	The course
The students	The clinical teachers
The students	Patients/clients
The clinical teachers	Patients/clients
The clinical teacher	Professional body

The clinical teacher needs to be as skilled and possibly even more skilled than the classroom teacher, as the former is expected to carry out two roles concurrently. Trying to meet the patients's needs, the student's needs and the needs/demands of the employing authority may sometimes create conflicts of interest. Nevertheless, as clinicians providing learning experience for students, clinical teachers are committed to carrying out these roles to the best of their ability. It is therefore necessary to consider the role, and the teaching and learning methods, more closely.

THE ROLE OF THE TEACHER WITH ADULT LEARNERS

Kolb (1984) in looking at education in general, defines three broad roles for the teacher to adopt in order to facilitate learning through experience:

1. To help participants to identify their own needs and to set their own goals.
2. To help participants to identify resources in response to individual need.
3. To help participants to create their own action plans based on need.

In broad terms these roles and aims are applicable to the role of the teacher in work experiences, such as clinical settings. However, in order to help clinicians to realize these roles, it is necessary to identify them more specifically.

Before doing this, it is worthwhile considering what is meant by 'teaching', a term used so frequently that we rarely pause to think what it means. Our own experiences as learners will influence our view of teaching. Probably our main experience of learning is based on a teaching approach designed for teaching children (pedagogy). For those who qualified before the 1980s this approach may have been dominant in their pre-registration course, especially if the course was externally set and examined by the professional body. Students on a pre-registration course, preparing for entry to a profession, are all adult learners for whom the characteristics of the pedagogical approach may not promote independent learning and therefore independent, autonomous professionals. The characteristics of the pedagogical approach include the following:

1. The teacher is responsible for deciding the content and pacing of the student's learning.
2. The experience and knowledge of the teacher is of major importance.
3. Learners are mainly oriented to a specific subject.
4. The teacher organizes and presents the material according to the logic of the subject matter.
5. External pressures such as competition, grades and the consequences of failure are the main motivations for learning.

This kind of teaching contrasts markedly with the student-directed (autonomous) approach which is characteristic of adult learning. Adult learning (androgogy) has very different characteristics from pedagogy and its use results in a radically different approach to the education process, (Knowles, 1975, 1980; Knowles *et al.*, 1984). Its main characteristics are:

1. As the individual learner matures, self-concepts change from independence to increasing independence and self-directedness.
2. Students' past experiences are taken fully into account in planning for individual learning needs, especially in the context of experiential learning.
3. Adult learners are ready to learn because they need to know or to do something to be more effective in some aspect of their life.
4. It is natural for adults to have a problem-oriented approach to learning. Relevant meaningful situations (e.g. clinical experiences) provide significant learning experiences.
5. Adults can be motivated to learn by internal rewards, such as increased self-esteem and a sense of accomplishment.
6. Adults will respond best to a collaborative relationship with the teacher, be it in the classroom or the clinic.

Boud (1988) also explores the way students become autonomous in their learning. He lists 16 characteristics, emphasizing: goal setting by the student; using teachers as guides and counsellors, rather than instructors; working collaboratively with others; undertaking additional self-directed work; self-evaluation and reflecting on the learning process. Bearing in mind the need to find an approach to clinical teaching for adult learners who are studying to enter a field of practice, it is now possible to consider the role of the clinical teacher.

THE CLINICAL TEACHER'S ROLE

In discussing 'role' with around 100 colleagues across the health professions, it has been valuable to try to reach a comprehensive list of the elements to be included in the clinical teacher's job. From talks with audiologists, chiropodists, dietitians, occupational therapists, orthoptists, physiotherapists, radiographers and speech therapists, during their attendance at clinical teaching courses, a fair consensus was reached on the following five elements:

- Managing the work experience provision
- Facilitating learning
- Extending knowledge and promoting its application
- Promoting skill development
- Promoting professionalism

It is not always easy to assign aspects of a job to particular headings, because there are overlaps and interconnections; however, each heading encapsulates useful concepts thought to be of importance by clinicians. An overall view of the job is depicted in Fig. 3.1. The items will now be discussed further; some will be returned to in more detail in later chapters.

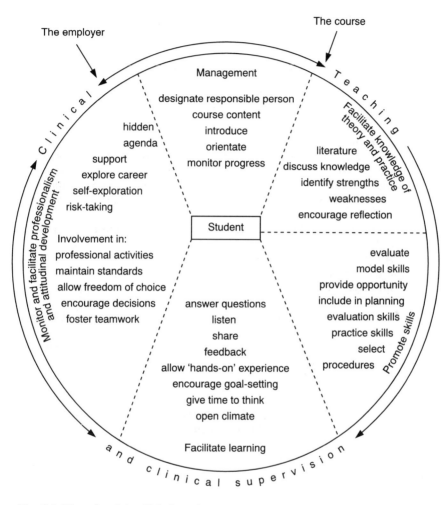

Fig. 3.1 The role of the clinical teacher.

Managing the work experience provision

Items under this heading are summarized in Box 3.2. It should always fall to one of the clinical team to liaise with the college placing the student and to set up provisions for receiving students. In many instances at the first level this will be the manager of the service or department. It is necessary for managers to be fully aware of the nature and demands of the placements in order that a managerial commitment to the time involved can be made.

Box 3.2 Managing the work experience

1. Managerial commitment of time.
2. Structure timetable, modify arrangements and experiences if necessary.
3. Plan case-load.
4. Prioritize the student's needs as they relate to the service provision.
5. Orientation to the work setting.
6. Communication with the course.
7. Explore and provide learning opportunities appropriate to the stage of the course the student has reached (course objectives for placement), including non-clinical activities, e.g. attending staff meetings.
8. Monitor the student's work-load, especially if the student is working with more than one clinician.
9. Allow the clinical teaching team to have enough time to teach the student as necessary.
10. Arrange access to a range of learning situations.
11. Provide a cohesive structure for clinicians and student(s).
12. Introduce the student to learning resources, e.g. library, equipment, other staff, as a knowledge resource.
13. Help the clinical teachers to be aware of their roles and responsibilities and support them in the role.
14. Appoint/designate a member of staff to have special responsibility for student teaching.

Experience from a range of health care professionals who have worked with students shows that it is very difficult to maintain a 'normal' case-load as well as carrying out effective clinical teaching, especially with a student who has little clinical experience. With more experienced students, and especially with those who are about to qualify, maintaining a full case-load may sometimes be possible. Occasionally there may even be an increase in case-load, for example, when the presence of a student enables a clinician to work with a group of patients or when students are able to carry out additional reviews, screening assessments or prescribed treatment sessions for patients needing intensive treatment. However, in most instances the case-load will tend to be reduced. Clinicians involved in taking students should be given the opportunity to make their commitment a positive choice, while managers will need to consider this as an essential part of their job and provide recognition and support.

Managing the programme

It will ususally be necessary for the person responsible for the setting up of the placement to arrange a programme for the student. This is particularly important when a student is to undertake an extended placement. The demands likely to be made on the student by each part of the experience needs to be seen as a whole and monitored. The possible content of the case-load should be planned as far as possible, and the needs of the student prioritized in the context of the service provision and the aims and objectives of the particular placement.

Contact with the course

It is hoped that the receiving district or department will have sufficient and appropriate contact with the student's course, so that receiving clinical teachers have information about the course as a whole and, in particular, about the stage of the course the student has reached. This can only be in broad terms, because although certain areas of the syllabus will have been covered, for each student the level of understanding will be different. However, although it is acceptable to expect a student to be prepared in areas they should have covered, it is not acceptable to expect them to have knowledge in areas which have not yet been addressed in college. There is a constant dilemma for course planners and receiving agencies, as students sometimes learn best in the classroom when the topic has been preceded by clinical experience; nevertheless, it is very difficult to ask clinicians to provide experience of cases where there is no preparation of the knowledge base. Careful guided observation is of immense value to student learning and is discussed in Chapter 5. It is a pity if clinical teachers will not let students see patients where they have not covered the condition theoretically, as a powerful learning opportunity will have been missed.

Clinical teachers from many fields complain that they do not have enough information for the courses they work with.

Learning opportunities

With the prerequisite information it should be possible to plan and provide learning opportunities appropriate to the stage of the course a student has reached. It may be necessary for the manager of the placement to arrange access to a variety of learning situations. These negotiations will be of particular importance when making provision for students to attend staff meetings, case conferences and to learn to work with other professionals. In some professions, experience outside the health authority, for example in educational and social services, will need to be set up.

Support and communication network

In the provision of learning opportunities for the student it is necessary to set up a coordinated cohesive structure for the department, the clinicians and the student. In this way all the participants will be aware of the programme for the student and their own role within it. It may be necessary to monitor the student's work-load either across college/clinic or across the different clinical settings. It is unfortunate if a student is seen as the particular responsibility of one clinician and not as a student member of the department or team.

Roles and responsibilities

It is the manager's responsibility to help clinicians to appreciate what their roles and responsibilities might be. Looking after the student and their programme is the kind of management job which can appropriately be devolved to a clinician, in the service, who has appropriate experience and is interested in clinical teaching. Ideally the staff member designated will see this area of work as part of the continuing education in their own career as well as being central to the future of the profession. It need not be the service or departmental manager who carries out this job. This 'key' clinical teacher provides an essential link with the college-base, the clinicians and the student. Prior to starting the placement, information should ideally be made available to the student about the service and clinics included in the placement. The provision of information packs for students will be considered further in the next chapter.

Receiving the student

The key clinical teacher will have a particular role in receiving the student and orientating them to the work setting. If the student is attending only one clinic/department the job can be undertaken by the clinicians there. The student's first impressions are, without doubt, very influential in forming their views and motivation about the experience that the placement has to offer. Clinicians are usually extremely hard-presssed, and it is, unfortunately, possible for students to be made to feel 'unwelcome' or 'in the way'. Preparing to receive the student will be considered further in the next chapter.

Facilitating learning

The list of functions perceived by clinical teachers as included in their 'role' is succinct and easily comprehensible; it is shown in Box 3.3. These points appear obvious and perhaps even easy to achieve when set out in a neat list. Some of them are of extreme importance in promoting student learning. The following should be noted as being of central importance:

Box 3.3 Facilitating learning

---

1. Answering questions.
2. Offering suggestions.
3. Facilitating desired behaviour.
4. Facilitating two-way discussions.
5. Encourage self-monitoring and evaluation.
6. Observation opportunities, provide guidelines for observation.
7. Learn from the student.
8. Listen to the student.
9. Give student time to reflect on what is happening and has happened.
10. Give student time to prepare.
11. Allow student to make mistakes in the confines of patient safety. Allow student to see your mistakes.
12. Encourage students to think for themselves.
13. Help the student to identify where they have reached in their learning.
14. Don't limit the student to your experience; allow student to make choices.
15. Help student to identify and set realistic goals.
16. Allow 'hands on' experience even when you think the task is complex.

- Providing opportunities and guidelines for observation
- Facilitating two-way feedback
- Helping the student to identify goals and to achieve them

These areas are of such importance that whole chapters or sections are devoted to them later in the book.

Extending knowledge and promoting its application

This aspect of the clinical teacher's job is central to clinical competence. Applying knowledge to practice is what we all do in our day-to-day work. It is particularly difficult to make accessible to the student knowledge and understanding which may be so deeply embedded in the practice of the clinician that they may not even be aware that it is there. This possession of tacit knowledge was discussed earlier.

Experienced clinicians will be aware that what was originally understood to be relevant to practice, may no longer be the most up-to-date and effective method. The student with more recent information may be aware of this. Everything that clinical teachers do is presumably aimed at helping the student to bring theory and practice together. However, the clinical teacher needs to help the student to access knowledge and apply it to a particular problem.

Box 3.4 Extending knowledge and facilitating knowledge application

1. Help the student to identify what he/she does/does not know.
2. Focus on the literature appropriate to practice.
3. Encourage the student to look up lecture notes.
4. Bring knowledge to relate to specific cases.
5. Consider the generality of theory in relation to the needs of particular patients.
6. Help the student to achieve a holistic view of the patient.
7. Try to bridge the gap between the classroom and clinic.
8. Provide opportunities for the students to use their own knowledge in assessment and treatment even if this knowledge is not shared by the clinical teacher.
9. Be aware of the progress and demands of the whole curriculum.
10. Encourage reflection through and on practice.

Box 3.5 Promoting skill development

Model and provide explanations on the use of skills and techniques, appropriate to the student's stage of professional development.

1. Provide opportunity for student to develop a range of skills:
   procedural, e.g. patient examination, diagnostic and treatment procedures;
   interactional and communicative;
   treatment techniques;
   problem-solving;
   administrative;
   managerial;
   multidisciplinary;
   clinical emergencies, first aid, etc.;
   surgical (chiropody/podiatry).
2. Help the student to become part of the team.
3. Foster skills in planning and evaluation.
4. Help student to establish a working relationship with relatives and carers, including opportunities to undertake domiciliary work
5. Opportunities to develop written communication skills:
   recording patient data;
   disseminating information;
   preparing reports;
   analysing and ordering information.

The student will be helped by being encouraged to: identify the knowledge they already have; refer back to the literature, lecture notes etc; look at recent journal articles; keep in view the needs of the patient as a whole; reflect on what they know and do. These ideas are listed in Box 3.4.

Promoting skill development

On the surface of professional work a number of skills can be observed. The student may have begun to get to grips with some of these in college, while others may be observed and tried out for the first time in clinic. The real setting is without doubt the best place to bring skills to a standard which is competent, safe and carried out with ease. The clinician will therefore play a central role in demonstrating techniques and skills and providing opportunity for students to use them. Box 3.5 lists some of the generic skills to be developed in all health professionals. These do not only include manual and psychomotor skills but include interpersonal, communicative, diagnostic and administrative abilities. Individuals will be able to identify skills specific to their own field.

Promoting professionalism

Professionalism includes both what we do on the surface and, just as importantly, the attitudes below the surface. As we have seen from the model in Chapter 1, these attitudes are the driving force for our professional practice. The role of the clinical teacher in helping the student towards their professional development is the area which is the least explicit, but probably the most pervasive, regarding future commitment to the professional field. It is here that covert messages will have a particularly strong influence; what is said by the teacher will not be influential if the student sees that practice does not match the theory. For example, if the clinician talks about team work, but does not in fact communicate effectively with other team members in, for instance, the rehabilitation unit, then the model of practice is likely to override anything the clinician or college tutor has said.

Teachers in the classroom and clinic therefore carry a brief to maintain standards of practice through modelling, exploring and explaining professional practice. The student will be aware of the clinician's commitment to clinical education, which in itself will act as a powerful role model. Box 3.6 provides some ideas for the clinical teacher to consider in fostering the development of professionalism. The exploration of **attitudes** is always a very sensitive area; some ideas to help facilitate attitudinal development are also suggested in Box 3.6, as professional and attitudinal development are closely linked.

The question of the clinical teacher needing to take a **pastoral role** in relation to the student is a difficult one and has already been touched on earlier

Box 3.6 Promoting professional and attitudinal development

1. Maintain and ensure standards of practice.
2. Check and review plans.
3. Enable student to become a decision-maker.
4. Model and provide explanations of standards of professional practice.
5. Explore the student's attitudes to people in the clinical situation.
6. Foster self- and time-management.
7. Balance patient and student needs.
8. Provide experience of the reality of work; 'politics'; budgeting, etc.
9. Help student to manage case-load.
10. Help student to deal with patient expectations.
11. Help student to develop to potential.
12. Encourage student self-exploration.
13. Analyse and explore career opportunities.
14. Encourage an awareness of the continuing education needs of staff.
15. Get to know the student; let the student get to know you.
16. Provide an open climate for the exchange of ideas, airing problems.
17. Assessing needs, being sensitive to needs.
18. Offering support, both academic and emotional.
19. Provide an enabling environment for student and course tutors.
20. Provide opportunity for risk-taking; mutual vulnerability involved in student/clinician/tutor/patient relationship.

in the discussion on being too much like a therapist. Students are adults and it is not the responsibility of teachers to monitor students' personal lives. It is inevitable that with the stress of being a learner some students are going to need the kind of support which is outside the role of the clinical teacher. It may be a particular problem where students are on an extended placement away from the college-base and peer support. Some students may be under the greatest stress when they attempt to be embryonic professionals and students at the same time. Being required to adopt both these roles within the same week is extremely demanding. Frequent and close contact needs to be maintained with the college tutor responsible for the student's progress.

A number of different tutoring arrangements may be found across courses. They are an important aspect of course management and monitoring, especially where students are learning to become professionals. From experience of many different tutoring arrangements, I believe the most helpful for the student and satisfying for staff is where each student has a tutor appointed to work with them throughout the duration of the course, or at least those parts of the course which include clinical work.

It is hoped that a full consideration of the role of the clinical teacher does not deter some clinicians from doing the job. Many of the skills are ones which we use in working with patients. For example: identifying needs, setting goals, facilitating feedback, working out the next step to take and facilitating desired behaviour. So also are the approaches to relating positively, fostering, facilitating, encouraging, providing and enabling, all within the day-to-day orientation of the health care worker. These are all components of professional competence and are therefore congruent with roles as clinical teachers.

Boyd-Webb (1984) identifies the phases of working with a student as the same as the phases of working with clients/patients. She identifies three phases: the beginning, characterized by anxiety, concern and expectation in the patient or student; the middle, where the student needs to be helped with maintaining a work focus and which is usually associated with a slump; the final one, which must involve the participants in review, summing up the process and identifying goals which still need to be reached.

It is evident that the clinician has the potential to be an effective clinical teacher. Many clinicians are already excellent teachers and will serve as role models for others. It is possible to believe, erroneously, that a competent clinician must necessarily be a competent clinical teacher. Obviously clinical competence is a prerequisite for teaching. Even for those with experience in teaching it is useful to stop and consider how the job may be approached, gathering ideas from colleagues in one's own and other fields. Clinicians who are recently qualified, for example in the last 2 years, have the potential to make good clinical teachers, especially as their own experience as learners in clinic is still easily accessible to them. They can benefit from the experience of others and the literature which is now available.

ANALYSING LEARNING STYLES

Teachers will remember clearly both students who they got along with well and others where the relationship was not so easy. Obviously there may be personality factors here, but in some instances it may be that difficulties arise in the teaching/learning context because the cognitive or learning styles of the student and clinical teacher may not be in agreement. These styles relate to the way individuals approach study, as well as the ways in which they think. Learning styles are related to personality and are nothing to do with an individual's intelligence. Professionals are committed to being lifelong learners. Personal experience of continuing education or learning for leisure may have helped to make us more aware of our own styles as learners. In the clinical situation, where teaching tends to take place on an individual basis, or sometimes with a small group of students, the teacher and learner(s) are brought together in close interface.

If the learning styles and the teaching styles of learner and teacher do not have some commonalities there may be the potential for tension.

Psychologists and educationalists examined learning styles and have identified different styles according to the researchers own theoretical orientation (school). Jobling (1987) provides a useful account of some of these as well as relating some of these views to physiotherapy and clinical teaching. An approach which a number of teachers of health students have found comprehensible, helpful and applicable both to teaching in the classroom and in the field of practice, is the learning styles described by Honey and Mumford (1986). Clinical teachers may find it interesting to obtain this and complete the learning styles' questionnaire. The questionnaire reveals the different ways in which people approach their learning and therefore how they may respond to different approaches to teaching, both in the classroom and in the clinic. In a college-based environment it is easier to provide a number of different learning opportunities, as described earlier. This gives all learners the opportunity to experience methods which they can respond to as individuals. However, with the practical focus of the clinical situation it may be easier to meet the needs of the learner who likes to try out ideas, likes to get on with things and act quickly, especially if the clinical teacher has a similar approach. It may not be so easy to meet the needs of the learner who likes to stand back, reflect and take time before acting. Although we all have a mix of characteristics, Honey and Mumford group the characteristics under four main learning styles:

- Activist
- Reflector
- Theorist
- Pragmatist

The learning styles' questionnaire poses 80 statements; some examples of these are:

No. 1   I have strong beliefs about what is right and wrong.
No. 16 I like to reach a decision carefully after weighing up many alternatives.
No. 32 I tend to be open about what I'm feeling.
No. 73 I do whatever is expedient to get the job done.

Scoring the questionnaire is plotted on an axis to show the mix of characteristics in the individual. The characteristics of the four styles are summarized in Box 3.7.

OTHER INFLUENCES ON TEACHING AND LEARNING IN CLINIC

Although learning styles are not related to personality, personality factors

Box 3.7 Description of learning styles. Adapted from Honey and Mumford (1986)

Activists:
> involve themselves fully, without bias in new experiences;
> enjoy the here and now, happy to be dominated by immediate experiences;
> open-minded, not sceptical;
> enthusiastic about anything new;
> dash in where angels fear to tread;
> like brainstorming problems;
> bored with implementation and longer-term consolidation;
> gregarious, involve themselves with others;
> seek to centre all the activities around them.

Reflectors
> like to stand back to ponder experiences, thoughtful;
> observe from many different perspectives;
> collect data, chew over before coming to conclusions;
> tend to postpone reaching conclusions;
> cautious, leave no stone unturned;
> prefer to take back seat in meetings and discussions;
> enjoy observing people in action;
> listen to others;
> adopt a low profile;
> have a slightly distant, tolerant, unruffled air.

Theorists:
> integrate observations into complex, logical theories;
> think problems through step-by-step;
> assimilate disparate facts into cohesive whole;
> tend to be perfectionists;
> like to anlayse;
> tend to feel uncomfortable with subjective judgments;
> tend to be detached, analytical and rational.

Pragmatists:
> keen on trying out ideas, theories and techniques;
> positively search out new ideas;
> like to experiment;
> like to get on with things and act quickly;
> tend to be impatient with lengthy open-ended discussions;
> essentially practical, like making practical decisions;
> respond to problems and opportunities as a challenge.

can, of course, affect those involved in the learning process. There are other less obvious factors which may be influential, including age, gender, cultural background and differences in qualifications. This last factor may be of particular significance in those fields which have changed from a diploma to a degree level of entry to the profession. The patient too will be important in the teaching/learning context. There may be very complicated scenarios in which the above influences are all caught up in the relationship of the student, clinical teacher and the patient.

Is the job purely technical?

Another strong influence on the way teaching is carried out in clinic is the way the work is envisaged. This relates to the points made earlier about the technical–interpersonal continuum of the work of the health professional. Even within one field there will be a range of stances along this continuum. If the professional field follows a very technical and prescriptive approach, necessary for the safety of patients, there may be a tendency to teach students in the same way, possibly not allowing students enough opportunity to think on their own. Alternatively, if the practitioner uses a lot of counselling there may be a tendency to deal with students in this way.

The interaction of student and teacher

However good the administrative arrangements are for student placements, the interpersonal aspects of the teacher–student relationship cannot be legislated for. Students and clinical teachers will get on in different ways and with different degrees of success in the teaching and learning experience. Where students work with only one clinician over a period of time, for example one day a week over a term, there is the potential for either an excellent or a negative learning experience. However, clashes of personality or learning style in this situation are potentially very damaging. Students would seem to be at an advantage if the placement provides opportunity for working with at least two clinical teachers concurrently. Students are understandably concerned that if they do not get on with a clinician this may influence their grading.

Direct and indirect styles in teaching

The exploration of learning styles through the completion of the learning styles' questionnaire, both by the student and the clinical teacher, as suggested earlier, provides a useful forum for students to talk bout their own approaches to learning and at the same time begin to see how the clinical teacher operates.

The teacher has particular responsibility to gain insight into the student's learning style, so that unrealistic expectations regarding the students behaviour are avoided. This means that clinical teachers also need to reflect on the predominant tendencies in their own approaches. Brasseur and Anderson (1983) investigated 'supervisory' styles through analysing and rating video-recordings of student–clinician conferences during the clinical placements of speech and language therapists.

Box 3.8 Direct and indirect teaching styles. Adapted form Brasseur and Anderson (1983)

Direct	Indirect
Dominated by the supervisor	More student-centered
High proportion of supervisor talking	Supervisor talks less; listens more.
Giving information	Supportive relationship
Giving opinions	Asks questions
Giving suggestions	Accepts and uses ideas
Gives criticisms	Reflects
	Summarizes student's ideas and feelings.
These styles lead to different behaviours in the learner	
Direct style leads to:	*Indirect style leads to:*
Supervisor control	Collaborative problem solving
Evaluation; supervisor as expert	
Student dependence	**Student independence**

Two main styles, **direct** and **indirect**, were identified. The characteristics of these styles are shown in Box 3.8. At some stage in their development students will require direction; this will be particularly true in their first clinical experience, when a new type of placement commences or a new client group is encountered. Clinical teachers need to be aware of the style they generally adopt and try to adjust according to the learning needs of a student, at any given stage of a course and of the student's own development. In general, students will need guidance and direction in the early stages of their work experience. When nearing qualification they should be encouraged to be self-determining and independent. Brasseur and Anderson also refer to the finding that 'supervisors', i.e. clinical teachers, often perceived their style as indirect, while the 'supervisees', i.e. the students, perceived it as direct. The research did suggest that there was no clear dichotomy between direct and indirect styles and that another instrument may be needed for the analysis of clinical teaching approaches. Nevertheless, the point has been well made that clinical teachers need to reflect on their own styles both as teachers and learners, in order to gain a better understanding of how these methods might affect the students.

Interpersonal communication

Pickering (1987) addressed the question of interpersonal communication between the student and clinical teacher in some depth. She explores the matter from a number of psychological and philosophical insights. She writes from the stance of an experienced clinical teacher trying to make sense of the complexities of the process. It is clear that she, even with much experience, regards the job of clinical teaching, or 'supervision' as she calls it, as a very complex one. She sees the interaction between clinical teacher and student as central and the most problematic aspect. Furthermore, like Boyd-Webb (1984) she sees the student–client relationship as having many similarities to the clinician's relationship with the student: 'I have needed help in making sense of my interactions with students and my students interaction with clients.' She discusses how Humanistic–Existential thought and the literature on interpersonal communication have helped her through the maze. Under the Humanistic–Existential heading she outlines the following topics.

- The validity of interpersonal perception
- The possibility of mutuality
- The potential for individual choice
- The relationship between behaviour and intent
- The importance of human growth and transformation
- The insistance of being holistic

It is beyond the scope of this book to discuss these topics further. Readers will find that Pickering's work enriches their understanding of their role as clinical teachers. She sees interpersonal communication as 'a critical dimension of the process' and focuses on three principles of interpersonal communication, which she finds have enhanced her understanding of clinical teaching interactions. These principles are:

1. **Communication occurs *between* not *in* individuals.** *Together* people create what happens; both teacher and learner are involved in this creation. This principle applied to clinical teaching means that there should be a focus on:
   (a) communicative behaviours and the roles of each person;
   (b) the meaning that communication appears to have for each person;

(c) the interpretations made by each person;

(d) patterns of communication behaviour over time;

(e) relational changes over time.

These points will have particular relevance in the situation where clinical teachers and college tutors are involved in providing feedback to students on their progress. Mismatch of meanings and different interpretations can easily occur on these occasions. This will be explored further in the section on feedback later in this volume.

2. **In a communication transaction, any action can be seen as the cause or effect, depending on the participant's perspective**. For example, a student may feel that a treatment plan had not been appropriate because the patient was uncooperative. The clinical teacher, on the other hand, may think that the objectives set for the client were at too high a level. Here the student needs to be helped to evaluate the effect of the treatment objectives on the patient.

    Similarly, a clinical teacher may be surprised that a student has not come prepared for a task set them. Whereas it could be possible that the teacher has not made it absolutley clear what was expected of the student. Whether or not the student can say to the clinician that they are not sure about what they were required to do, may relate to the clinical teacher's style, or the student's style but could also relate to lack of time, to presumptions, etc.

3. **Individuals do not exist alone, but live and function within a social network of meaning**. Meanings that are clear to experienced clinical teachers may not be clear to the learner. In running clinical teaching courses across health care professions it has become evident that we all have our own 'social networks of meaning'. The experience of learning alongside other health care colleagues through multidisciplinary, continuing education courses, on appropriate topics such as counselling, management, communication skills, quality assurance, audit, assessment of competence and clinical teaching, is important in learning to make our knowledge and understanding accessible to others. We are usually so caught up in our own professional world that we are not aware of how inaccessible it may be to others. Furthermore, students may bring new meanings from their more recent theoretical studies. They should be encouraged to share these with the clinical teachers. Some departments may even encourage students to present new methods to the whole clinical team, providing a wonderful model of the need for lifelong professional learning.

Pickering lists another nine principles which she sees as important. They continue as follows:

4. Communication is a process not a thing.

5. Communication is circular not linear.

6. Communication involves the total personality.
7. Communication is complex.
8. In a transaction an individual cannot fail to communicate.
9. Meanings, ideas and information are conveyed through a variety of message systems, of which oral language is only one.
10. Messages have more than one level of meaning.
11. Transactions involve individuals at multiple levels of perspective.
12. The self is created and maintained through interpersonal transactions.

Clinical teachers and students need to be aware of their role in the communication process. The development of good interpersonal skills is germane to the work of all health care professionals. It is therefore an area which should be addressed in the curriculum in college, prior to the student undertaking work experience. The student's interpersonal skills will affect interaction with both clients and clinical teachers. It is of little value for students to possess relevant knowledge and technical skills if these cannot be applied, because the student is unable to carry out the first phase of the clinical process of setting up an appropriate relationship with the client and the team. This factor may vary in importance according to the nature of the clinical practice. For example, an X-ray of a patient can be obtained if the student carries out what is required with 'bad grace', but the student dietitian may not be able to proceed if a patient is unwilling to provide dietary information. Again, if a speech and language therapy student cannot set up a rapport with a child to encourage the child to speak, it may not be possible to collect speech data for analysis. Clinical teachers should check with the course on what has been covered on interpersonal skill development, prior to placement.

Clinical teachers need to ensure that communication skills with students are as effective as communication skills with clients. Whatever has been covered in the classroom, nothing can replace the strong role model presented by the clinical teacher.

FOLLOW-UP ACTIVITIES

1. Make a list of the skills students needed to acquire. Divide the list into (i) generic to all health professionals; (ii) specific to your own field.
2. If you work in a clinical teaching team, discuss the role as outlined in this chapter with your colleagues. Develop a model which best represents the clinical teacher's role in your own field.
3. Consider the characteristics of the Honey and Mumford (1986) learning styles (Box 3.7). Consider which characteristics most fit your own style.

4. Obtain a learning styles' questionnaire, complete it yourself and get a student to complete it. Compare your style with the student's style and the possible consequences.
5. Check with the course regarding students' college-based opportunities for the development of communication skills.

REFERENCES

Boud, D. (1988) *Developing Student Autonomy*, 2nd edn, Kogan Page, London; Nicols Publishing Co., New York.

Boyd-Webb,. (1984) From social work practice to teaching the practice of social work. *Journal of Education for Social Work*, **20**, no. 3, 55–7.

Brasseur, J.A. and Anderson, J.L. (1983) Observed Differences between Direct, Indirect and Direct/Indirect Video-taped supervisory conferences. *Journal of Speech and Hearing Research*, **26**, 344–55.

Hawkins, P. and Shohet, R. (1989) *Supervision in the Helping Professions*, Open University Press, Milton Keynes.

Honey, P. and Mumford, A. (1986) *The Manual of Learning Styles,* Printique, Berkshire.

Jobling, M. (1987) Cognitive Styles: Some Implications for Teaching and Learning. *Physiotherapy*, **73**, no. 7, 335–8.

Kolb, D. (1984) *Experiential Learning*, Prentice Hall, New Jersey.

Knowles, M.S. (1975) *Self-directed Learning: A guide for learners and teachers*, Association Press, New York.

Knowles, M.S. (1980) *The Modern Practice of Adult Education: from Pedagogy to Androgogy, Cambridge Books, New York.*

Knowles, M.S. et al. (1984) *Androgogy in Action*, Jossey-Bass, San Francisco.

Marson, S. (1990) Creating a climate for learning. *Nursing Times*, **86**, no. 17, 53–5.

Pickering, M. (1987) Interpersonal communication and the supervisory process, in Crago, M.B. and Pickering, M. (eds) *Supervision in Human Communication Disorders*, Little Brown & Co, Boston.

Stengelhofen, J. (1991) *A Cross Professional approach to Cinical Supervisors Courses*, Unpublished paper, Health Care Professions Educational Forum Study Day.

4

Preparing for working with students in clinic

INTRODUCTION

This chapter is designed to help readers prepare themselves and their department for receiving and working with students in their place of work. Particular attention is paid to the start of the student placement and the identification of objectives which can be met within the clinical teacher's own clinical setting.

However well the classroom has prepared students for practice, through the use of teaching methods designed to bridge the classroom–clinic gap, when students go to their first placement they will almost always experience some degree of anxiety. Indeed, one might feel somewhat concerned if they did not. Health care student are not alone in this experience. Boyd-Webb (1984) identified anxieties in social work students. The anxieties she listed are equally applicable to health students:

1. Anxiety about what would be expected of one.
2. Concern about interacting with the helping or teaching person and about whether this will be a relationship of mutual positive regard and respect.
3. Worry about one's performance or quality of participation compared to others.
4. Concern that the teacher will show preference or take sides.
5. Hope that the expectations for help or learning will be realized.

Apart from the first one, these anxieties are difficult to address prior to the placement. Course documentation should in broad terms cover 'what will be expected of one' as this presumably relates to the elements of competence (expressed in the course objectives), which the student is expected to develop during a given period, as well as which of the elements will be assessed. It will also relate to the types of cases and settings a student will experience.

Students are likely to be more anxious if they are unsure of what is going to happen. The more students are encouraged to be independent about their own learning responsibilities, the more they are likely to be able to handle anxieties, as they will feel more in control of what is happening. It is also reassuring for them to know that it is usual for students to feel anxious about going to clinic.

PREPARING THE STUDENT FOR THE WORK EXPERIENCE

We have already seen that students on different courses, even within the same profession, have varying patterns of work experience. Students going to a clinic on the college site for the first practice placement, do not have as big a step to take as the student going away from the geographical locality of the course on a placement. Students going away from college may have to leave the peer group and even go to live in another locality, while the student undertaking a concurrent weekly placement will return to the support of the peer group and college tutors for the rest of the week. Different course designs make different demands on students. This inevitably impinges upon the relative demands made on placement agencies and clinical teachers. Several of the professions arrange extended placements away from the college-base. Students need particularly careful preparation before such placements. The following approaches, which may be used in college, should help to ease the student into the real experience:

1. Attendance at clinical demonstrations.
2. Training in observation skills.
3. Arranging for students beginning clinical practice to observe another student, at a later stage of the course, treating patients.
4. Visits to other settings to have interface with the public, but not in the clinician/patient role.
5. Problem-solving activities related to cases.
6. Interpersonal skill-development exercises.
7. Case discussion through video examples, etc.
8. Role play.
9. Patient simulation exercises.
10. Discussions with students at later stage of the course on their placement experiences.
11. Raising students consciousness of the knowledge and skill they have acquired since beginning the course.

A HANDBOOK FOR STUDENTS AND CLINICAL TEACHERS

Tutors in college need to maintain a balance between telling the students too much about the placement (thus raising their anxiety) and not telling them enough. A good deal of information can be provided in written form, perhaps in a handbook, as anxious students may well forget what has been said to them in briefing sessions in college. Clinical teachers should find out if the course they are working with provides a handbook and, if so, secure a copy. This handbook should have been prepared in consultation with the receiving agencies. The clinical practice handbook can therefore be prepared as a resource for both the students and clinical teachers.

Box 4.1 provides suggestion for the contents of a clinical teacher/student handbook.

Box 4.1 Suggested content for student/clinician handbook

---

1. An outline of the whole curriculum and how the placements are arranged within it.
2. Aims of each stage of placement.
3. Case-load appropriate to the stage of the course.
4. Clinical settings appropriate to the different stages of the course.
5. Competencies to be assessed at the end of each placement.
6. Requirements for case studies, diaries, log books, etc. at each stage.
7. Methods of assessment, including pro formas, criteria for grades. The clinical teacher's role in assessment.
8. Range of clinical test/assessment procedures to be used if appropriate to the clinical field.
9. Nature, aims, number and timing of tutor visit to students during each placement.
10. Financial arrangements: transfer of grant, travel expenses.
11. Reference lists from course at various stages of student progress.

   Note that the handbook should be provided for each clinician working with the student, as well as a copy for the student.

AN INFORMATION PACK FOR STUDENTS

Some courses prepare detailed information on each clinical setting used regularly for student placement. These documents contain information on departments and units used by the course, including the types of patients seen and treatments routinely offered; resource guidelines for each placement; travel information; names of staff; telephone numbers; assessment pro formas; etc. This kind of format is appropriate when a course works regularly with a fairly small number of clinical settings; it may not be practicable for some other courses.

For example, some courses may work with as many as 60 different health authorities, while in each district students may work in different clinical settings. In this instance it would be valuable for each identifiable receiving unit to produce its own information pack or leaflet. This could be done clinic-by-clinic, by service (e.g. services for adults) or could be generated by the health authority, trust or school. Information from each clinic needs to be brief and should be regularly updated. It could easily form part of a more comprehensive package, for use in the service as a whole.

Box 4.2 gives suggestions for the contents of an information pack for students. In order not to overload the student it might be helpful to divide the information into two categories: (i) information for the student to have before going to the placement, and (ii) information which will be needed during the placement and which should be written down as a reference source. This should be given to the student during the induction period.

An examination of such packages suggests that in addition to them being used for students they can also be valuable for many other purposes, for example when visitors come to the department.

The inclusion in some of the packs of the controversial area of terminology is interesting. This in fact could provide a useful forum for discussion with the student, to establish how the clinician's definitions might differ from the student's own, learnt in college or on an earlier placement. The inclusion of the clinical library list, which might also give information on the postgraduate medical library, gives an important message about the kind of learning experience involved. The provision of the pro forma for the student to give feedback on the placement experience could be used to great value.

For students going on extended placements, away from their base, information on accommodation will be required, while information on local social activities will be reassuring. Other types of information will need to be conveyed to the student at an early point in the placement. It may still be done best in written form, backed up by discussion to clarify and point up important areas. The following points are suggested for some of the contents:

- Access to information, e.g. case notes
- Health and safety
- Security and emergency procedures
- Sickness procedures
- Ordering transport
- Procedures for patient data collection (e.g. hospital codes, activity codes, etc.)

Health authorities will have their own checklists used for new staff, which will provide useful guidelines to clinical teachers on the kind of material to be covered; some of this may be appropriate for student use.

Box 4.2 Information for student

A. **Information made available before placement**. To serve as valuable orientation material prior to arrival.

1. Maps of locality.
2. The size and nature of the population in the locality.
3. Role of the profession, as seen by the receiving agency.
4. Organization and size of the service, including the staffing structure and clinical locations.
5. Nature of case-load and types of treatment routinely offered (particularly relevant to some fields and some placements which may be procedurally focused).
6. Liaison with other disciplines.
7. Library provision including the need for an introductory letter from academic institution.
8. Staff profiles.
9. Terminology.
10. What to bring to the placement, e.g. equipment, literature. Guidelines on dress.
11. Social and sporting facilities.

B. **Information to be covered early on in the placement**. The following topics will need to be covered, but are perhaps best left until the student has arrived. It is advisable that they are in written form to serve as a reminder to the student and to discourage enthusiastic staff from overloading students with too much information during initial briefing sessions.

1. Health and safety regulations.
2. Layout of workplace; toilets, changing facilities, coffee, lunch, etc.
3. Guidelines on confidentiality.
4. Advice sheets on 'golden rules' on procedures.
5. Record-keeping, including use of computing, including patient, hospital and activity codes, etc.
6. Liaison with voluntary organizations.
7. Photocopying facilities.
8. Opportunities for visits to other departments, units, etc.
9. Form to be completed at the end of the placement for the student to provide feedback on the experience.

Some placements also include worksheets in their information packs for students, with questions about various aspects of the service. This is an excellent way for making the student active in learning, as well as helping them to reach a real understanding of how a service operates. Some courses in fact expect students to focus particularly on the service as a whole as an objective for the placement.

When information packs are provided they become a long-lasting resource. It also ensures that all the important points are on record for students to refer to and that the student has not been overwhelmed by the information being passed on orally at an early stage in the placement. Word processing facilities make it easy to update the information.

However much information colleges and health authorities provide, students will still pose some questions which are very difficult to answer in a written format. Here are some examples:

- What will my role be?
- What will they expect of me?
- How will I know how I'm doing?
- What will the clinicians be like?
- Who do I go to with problems?
- Am I expected to know everything?
- How will I know what tests to use?
- What if I have too much work to do?

Some of these questions might be more easily tackled in discussion with the student at the beginning of the placement.

The question **what will the clinician be like?** may be eased by the provision of short pen sketches of staff, so that at least the name rings a bell and the student is aware of a clinician's particular interests, thus easing the first meeting. If a student is going away from the college-base on an extended placement, the start may be helped by receiving a welcoming letter. The three letters in Boxes 4.3, 4.4 and 4.5 are all in very different styles, but each appropriate in their individual way. It is a good idea to draft one to fit your own situation. As some of the points in these examples may raise the student's anxiety level, it might be appropriate just to provide a map and time of arrival, saying that the first morning will be set aside for questions and discussion. Such letters could also be used to remind students that they need to bring certain material/equipment to the placement. I like the list of journal articles to be included in the letter in Box 4.3; this gives the student something specific they can do to prepare themselves for the experience.

Some courses encourage students to write to the placement to intro-duce themselves; this is good practice and in line with the adult learning experience. The student should be encouraged, by the college tutor to include in the letter, relevant course/college information and personal details such as on health, handicapping or other personal information which may affect work, attendance, etc. This is reflected in the letter in Box 4.4.

Box 4.3 Content of letter of welcome to orthoptic student: Child Development Centre, Yorkshire Region

On your first few visits to the Child Development Centre your main role will be to observe, help in play situations with children, and get toys and equipment for the vision group.

When observing you may find it helpful to refer back to the checklists, noting especially the child's eye contact with people and toys, the relationship with the parent, response to other people, head posture, hand/eye coordination.

You may find the following articles helpful in relation to the work in the Child Development Centre;..

You will probably see some very handicapped babies and children while you are here. Also there will be very confidential discussions with parents and other professionals. Some parents may become distressed. If you find these things upsetting please talk about this with me, fellow students and the orthoptic teachers in college. It may help you to remember that patients are children with disabilities – each child has their own personality, even the most disabled. Try to seek this out and play and assess them at their level – you will find their response rewarding.

You will also note how much longer is needed to assess each child and talk to parents than is needed for usual orthoptic appointments. The approach to parents will also be different. Families with disabled children are disabled families, so not only the whole child has to be viewed on assessment, but the whole family situation. Social workers provide counselling to parents but therapists often need to listen and advise too.

During the year you will be able to spend time with other therapists in the team and they will discuss the main aspects of their work with you. The close links between their interests and the orthoptists will be very clear.

I hope that you enjoy your visits. Do not hesitate to ask questions and discuss problems – I am here to help you.

Box 4.4 Content of letter of welcome to speech and language therapy student: Hounslow and Spelthorne Speech and Language Therapy Service

We hope that you will enjoy your placement with us.

The attached information pack is designed to help you understand how our service works, what we have to offer you while you are with us and what we expect from your college. Please read it before your first day. We will go over any queries you may have when we see you, but if you have any urgent questions you can phone me on _____.

Please confirm that you are starting your placement with us on _____. We suggest that you arrive at _____. Before your arrival it would help us in planning your time if you could send us some information about yourself. We would like to know a little about your background, your academic interests, previous clinical experience and your objectives for this placement.

We look forward to meeting you. Involvement in student training is an enjoyable and stimulating, as well as a time-consuming experience for us. We expect to learn from you as well as with you and we hope that you will be happy with us.

Box 4.5 Content of letter of welcome to student in chiropody: Portsmouth and South East Hampshire Chiropody Service

In the near future you will be joining in the nail operations team at this hospital for a day. I am sending you some information about our district and department which I hope you may find of interest.

The clinic starts at 9 a.m. with the first patients booked for 9.15 a.m. The morning session is held in the Accident and Emergency Department. Please be on time and come with a clean uniform and badge.

At lunch time we usually eat together in the staff restaurant. Meals and snacks are available from about 70 pence, please feel free to join us.

The afternoon session starts at 1.10 p.m. the first patients are booked at 1.15 p.m. We are usually finished and packed up by 4.30 p.m.

I have enclosed an information pack for you, together with a map. If you have a car, parking may be a problem, and it may be in your best interests to use the train; the clinic is only 10 minutes walk from the station.

If you have any questions I am available on the above number on Monday and Tuesday afternoons.

We look forward to meeting you in the near future.

INFORMATION FROM THE COURSE ON STUDENT PROGRESS

Many institutions are not willing to provide the receiving placements with details of a student's in-course progress (personal and academic). This provision of information is thought to be unwise in the context of the findings on teacher expectations and student learning. It is considered safest to regard all students as equal, when they are received for work experience, therefore college should provide information on only the student's college and practical experiences to date. The only additional information which should be provided would relate to health or handicapping conditions which may have particular significance for the clinical setting or the role a student is to undertake. However, this information should only be given with the permission of the student concerned and would best be done in the introductory letter from the student him/herself.

Exceptions to not passing on information about a student's progress would be made when a student is undertaking additional clinical work, due to failure or referral. It is up to individual student's to make known to the clinicians any information on personal matters and academic progress if they wish to do so. Some students who do not do particularly well in college feel much more at ease in the clinical setting. This may have a positive effect on their learning and may well accelerate their grasp of the knowledge base, which teachers on the course may previously have considered to be weak.

Hanscombe (1986) explored teacher expectations in relation to the development of professionalism in physiotherapy students. She looked at the self-concepts of both the clinical teachers and the students. She found that there was a relationship between students' achievements and teachers' self-concepts. She also found that the curriculum, including that part which happens in clinic, does not enhance the self-construct of the weaker student as much as that of the good student. Furthermore, students appear to have an accurate picture of the way teachers judge them.

Where students have already undertaken practical experience on their course, they should ideally have identified their own needs and goals for their further development. It is beneficial if these needs and goals are shared with the clinical teachers in the new placement. Setting and achieving goals will be considered later.

STUDENT ANXIETIES

In addition to the general anxieties usually experienced by students, some of the anxieties arise because of the nature of a specific setting. Spowart (1987), researched and described the feelings of physiotherapy students facing 'the transition from the relative safety of the first year to the harsh realities of the first clinical placement in the second year'. Thirty physiotherapy students were asked to complete anonomously the sentence: 'my biggest fear about treating surgical patients is. . . .' Their responses are shown in Box 4.6. Spowart makes the point that the surgical placement may not be the most stress-provoking situation with which the physiotherapy student is faced. Intensive care units, coronary care units and cardiothoracic surgical units are cited as being more stress provoking. The physical aspects of these situations are without doubt potentially extremely stressful for students.

Students' anxieties may not only be in direct proportion to the physical aspects or life-threatening implications of a situation. Students in other professional groups may experience high levels of anxiety and fear about working in certain contexts. Examples might be of working with mentally or physically handicapped individuals, where the unknown factors, especially in relation to a student's own responses, makes them extremely fearful. They will also be fearful about dealing with individuals who are violent. Clinicians will be aware that what is a normal day-to-day working situation for professionals may be anxiety-provoking for others, especially

Box 4.6 Student anxieties. Adapted from Spowart (1987)

1. **Worries related to knowledge:**
   knowing: where to start;
              what to do with the patient;
   not knowing what to do;
   not being able to cope with the condition and the consequences;
   not being sure of the best treatment for a particular patient.
2. **Worries related to death/cardiac:**
   fear of making the patient's condition worse;
   if the patient dies and I won't know what to do, I'll feel responsible;
   fear of being left to deal with the cardiac arrest or haemorrhage;
   fear of not being able to cope if complication arises.
3. **Worries related to concern for patient:**
   doing the wrong thing and making the condition worse;
   patient suffocation due to mucus;
   pulling out drip or tube while mobilizing patient and not knowing where
   to stick it again;
   making the patient's scar open up by asking him to exercise..
4. **Worries concerning student's own reactions:**
   'I'll be sick on the patient';
   fear of panicking if anything goes wrong;
   fear of fainting.

students and patients. Clinical teachers need to acknowledge openly the possibility of these anxieties, thus signalling to students that these are usual and acceptable. It may be helpful to get the student to identify their anxieties more specifically so that they can be discussed and rationalized.

STUDENT EXPECTATIONS

It may be very helpful to try to ascertain what expectations, and anxieties, students have about their placement. Some useful questions for clinical teachers to ask, perhaps in a written format, might be:

1. What expectations do you have of your clinical training?
2. What expectations do you have of your clinical teacher/supervisor?
3. What do you think your supervisor/teacher might expect of you?
4. What do you think you are good at?
5. What do you think you need to work at?

Box 4.7 Expectations a student nurse has of a clinical teacher

---

Third year

1. A kind and friendly manner.
2. Approachable.
3. Knowledgeable.
4. Takes an interest in students/learners.
5. Patience and tolerance.
6. Creates a learning environment, i.e. teaching suitable/relevant subjects, at a level appropriate for each individual.

Box 4.8 Examples of students expectations of themselves

Two third-year students:

'Hope to increase confidence and experience working with a variety of patients and conditions. Would like supervision to decrease gradually and take on increasing responsibility, but for support to be available when necessary. I want to reinforce theoretical knowledge I've picked up in college by putting it into practical use. At present working with amputees for 6 weeks. Present supervision working alongside OT, but given increasing independence in routine matters, and beginning to take on a case-load of patients'.

'Six-week placement at school for physically handicapped children. I am working with two OT's and teachers and doing individual sessions on my own. I have completed one week. I hope to be able to function totally independently at the end of my 6 weeks, but I don't think this is possible because it is too short a time to gain all the skills needed. I hope to build up on this placement when on my next and then fulfil my main expectations'.

Student three:

1. Practice techniques learned in college.
2. Be allowed to practice skills in those areas I am not confident.
3. Get a wide range of experience and learn as much as possible.
4. To be allowed to formulate my own aims of treatment and methods, but to be able to discuss them if required.
5. To have feedback and positive criticism.

---

6. What are you concerned about following your previous placement?
7. What expectations do you have of yourself?

What students say about their expectations may give useful insight into their anxieties and whether or not they are being realistic about the placement aims. I liked the views of one first-year student; 'A high quality of experience and knowledge. Good relations with staff and learners. The ability to teach and keep things understandable – not just drone on in abbreviations and large Latin words'. Box 4.7 gives another example of what students expect of their clinical teacher, while the examples in Box 4.8 focus on what the students themselves expect to do.

AIMS FOR THE STUDENT IN YOUR CLINICAL SETTING

Providing students with a clear picture of the clinical setting and the cases within that setting, as well as identifying the learning outcomes for them, appropriate to the stage of the course, will be a way of reassuring them that they will not be required to do anything or take responsibility beyond what can legitimately be expected. Boxes 4.9–4.15 show examples of aims/learning outcomes from a range of settings from the professional groups with which we are concerned. Some of these are expressed in general terms, while others are expressed in specific behavioural objectives. Make sure you study the examples from *all* the professional groups. This will help you to identify ideas which are the most useful to your own working situation. Box 4.9(b) (chiropody/podiatry) achieves a nice balance between the specifics of a field and an understanding of health provision as a whole. While 4.9(a) concentrates on the assessment of an individual patient/client, including some elements which are of general importance to student learning, for example 'demonstrate a willingness to accept constructive criticism'.

The dietetics examples – Boxes 4.10(a) and (b) – show aims and objectives related to specialisms in clinical practice.

Box 4.11(a) encompasses a wide range of skills to be developed by the occupational therapy student, including verbal and written communication skills. The final placement example from occupational therapy – Box 4.11(b), demonstrates the level of independence required in a student's final placement. The interesting words are; 'determine, analyse, independently', and 'philosopy and practice of occupational therapy'.

Box 4.12(a) stresses the development of the orthoptics student's diagnostic skills, then leading the student on to being able to discuss management options. It is good to see the heading 'application of theory to practice'

Box 4.9 Aims for identified settings: chiropody

(a) Elizabeth Carpenter, Coventry

Patients eligible for treatment refer themselves or are referred by a GP, district nurse or a consultant. The appointment system is known as the self-referral system. The patients are asked to refer themselves back for treatment when they are in need of it. They are given an assurance that an appointment will be available within 14 days of the request.

Staffing

District Chief II, Chief III, Chief IV – 2, Senior I Senior II – 6, part time root-care assistants – 6. Private chiropodists do some part-time contract work.

Nail surgery assessment clinic

This is a special clinic to which patients have been referred having initially been seen by other chriopodists. Patients are then assessed as to whether or not they would benefit from nail surgery and the urgency of treatment is assessed.

Student aims

1. To understand the principles on which nail surgery assessment is based.
2. To learn to administer the assessment.
3. To develop the appropriate attitude to patients.

(b) L. Philpott, Dudley Health Authority

Aims for the student

1. To provide opportunity to observe several different practitioners working.
2. To liaise and communicate with a variety of different health care professionals.
3. To gain an insight into how these different professionals work.
4. To gain an understanding of the work in several different areas within the chiropody profession, e.g.: paediatrics, nail surgery, biomechanical assessment, orthotics laboratory.
5. To be able to understand the workings of a prescription-based orthotic service.
6. To be aware of different referral systems.
7. To gain an understanding of the different roles of health care professionals and their relevance to chiropody.
8. To begin to gain a basic understanding of assessment techniques.
9. To begin to gain an understanding of the formulating of a treatment plan.
10. To begin to learn to be able to categorize patients into levels of priority or risk.

Box 4.9 (continued)

(c) Aims for a second year student attending the department one day a week for a term (approximately 10 weeks), Southampton and South West Hampshire Health Authority

Aim:

Patient assessment.

Objectives:

At the completion of the term the student will be able to:

1. take a comprehensive personal, medical and problem history;
2. perform a clinical examination of: footwear, motor function, sensory function, joint function, skin structure, circulation;
3. evaluate presenting lesion and symptomatology;
4. write up history and examination;
5. construct a treatment plan from the information acquired;
6. understand the social and environmental circumstances of the patient and how they relate to the prognosis;
7. maintain the dignity of the patient in all clinical situations;
8. demonstrate a willingness to accept constructive criticism;
9. recognize areas of weakness and demonstrate an ability to remedy them;
10. analyse a problem in chiropodial care and suggest a project to investigate it.

---

in Box 4.12(b), as one of the work experience aims. Again the student's ability to discuss is seen as important.

The physiotherapy examples – Box 4.13(a) and (b) – include the specialism of paediatrics and the elderly, there is an emphasis here on 'recognize, describe, analyse and discuss', all very important skills for the developing professional.

The radiography examples Boxes 4.14(a), (b) and (c) – relate to specialism within the field. It seems to be helpful to divide the aims under 'care of the patient' and 'techniques'. It is so easy for students to get caught up in what they themselves have to do, that they forget what is happening to the patient.

The examples in Box 15(a) to (c) speech and language therapy, shows how it may be necessary to couch the aims in a wider context. In the example of a student working in a school for children with learning difficulties, the role of the speech and language therapist is included as one part of the total experience. Breaking down the learning aims for the student into:

Box 4.10 Aims for identified settings: dietetics, Leeds General Infirmary

---

(a) Acute service dietetics: a mix of inpatient and outpatient work; 9-week placement.

Aim:

On completion the student will be able to participate, with supervision, in the provision of acute service dietetics.

Objectives:

1. To carry out the tasks required to ensure a patient receives their correct diet.
2. To record accurately appropriate details on the record cards, inpatient notes, in letters, etc.
3. To show knowledge of:
    (a) how biomechanical parameters and medical history relate to the disease state;
    (b) theory of dietary treatment of usual acute service problems, e.g. diabetes, altered fat, etc.;
    (c) nutritional content of food, etc.
4. To make dietary assessments based on meal patterns, dietary recall, food records as appropriate.
5. To interview patients or their proxy unsupervised.
6. To establish working relationships with other staff involved in patient care, i.e., nurses, doctors, cooks, etc.
7. To provide patient education, with the support of diet sheets, and a qualified dietitian.
8. To participate in evaluating a patient's progress.

(b) Student training in renal dietetics

Overall aims:

1. Student will have insight into renal dietetics and the role of the renal dietitian.
2. Be competent to give dietary advice for the dietary problems that may be encountered in any hospital.

Objectives:

1. To demonstrate basic physiological, medical, pharmaceutical and nutritional knowledge of renal disease.
2. To be able to relate clinical condition and biochemical results to dietary treatment.
3. To demonstrate the ability to give appropriate dietary advice:
    low protein
    low protein, low salt;
    low protein, low salt, low potassium;
    nephrotic syndrome.

Box 4.11 Aims for specified settings: occupational therapy,: Linda Finlay, St James's Hospital, Leeds

---

Aims:
1. Assessment techniques:
   carry out independently and appropriately an initial and a progress interview, semi-structured interview;
   use self-rating questionnaire in collaboration with patients, e.g. role checklist, social skills questionnaire.
2. Engage patients in occupational therapy:
   build up appropriate professional relationships;
   encourage at least one patient to attend occupational therapy;
   introduce self and explain occupational therapy, and therapy aims to patient.
3. Plan and lead an activity group independently:
   either a task- or socially-oriented group;
   appropriately co-lead a more psychodynamically orientated group.
4. Verbal reporting:
   report back appropriately on patient's performance in sessions;
   report clearly on patient's progress with OT at a ward round.
5. Written reporting:
   write at least one of the following reports: home visit, initial assessment, progress;
   write letters to referring agents and patients;
   write up appropriately patient's progress, at the end of session.

Objectives for a final placement:
By the end of this placement the student will be able to:
1. Demonstrate ability to determine the needs and abilities of patients, applying appropriate assessment techniques.
2. Demonstrate the ability to vary personal communication skills and OT approaches appropriately in professional relationships with patients.
3. Analyse the contribution of the OT process.
4. Carry out independently and appropriately the OT process.
5. Demonstrate attitudes and behaviours appropriate to the philosophy and practice of OT.
6. Demonstrate appropriate communication skills for interprofessional communication.

---

administrative, liaison with staff and carers, and professional development, helps to make explicit what the student is required to achieve. I like the aims which say 'gain experience' suggesting that this experience is part of an ongoing cumulative process. It is good to see an example of aims expressed

Box 4.12 Aims for identified settings: orthoptics, Leeds School of Orthoptics, Leeds General Infirmary

---

(a) Overall aims of clinical work

  1. To be able to diagnose all types of squint.
  2. To diagnose mechanical and neurogenic motility disorders.
  3. To understand the reasons for using special diagnostic techniques, e.g. Hess/Field of BSV/Uniocular fixation.
  4. Accurately carry out all levels of orthoptic diagnostic tests.
  5. Classify conditions from test results.
  6. Discuss options of management.
  7. Be aware of the outcomes of management by follow-up of cases.
  8. Evaluate the effect of different surgical procedures by seeing pre- and post-operative cases.
  9. Apply special techniques to deaf, handicapped, very young and very old patients.
 10. Communicate information to patients/parents/colleagues.

(b) Extract from aims for orthoptics students, Spring Term, second year.
Diagnostic skills:

  1. Diagnose and classify all types of concomitant strabismus unaided.
  2. Diagnose isolated muscle palsies with assistance;
  3. Diagnose classical mechanical deviations in cooperative patients.
  4. Suggest whether incomitant deviation is congenital or acquired.
  5. Describe development of muscle sequelea.

Application of theory to practice:

  1. Relate neuro-anatomy to muscle palsy.
  2. Know muscle sequelae and and laws of innervation.
  3. Understand aetiology of mechanical deviations.

Management skills:

  1. Know indications for conservative and surgical treatment.
  2. Measure and apply Fresnels prisms to selected cases.
  3. Discuss types of surgery available.
  4. Actively take part in clinical duties.
  5. Communicate effectively with medical staff and patients/parents.

---

under the heading 'Potential for student learning'; is this perhaps a more realistic heading?

Box 4.16 is an example of more general professional aims. Although these were set up by one discipline, it is clear that they have general application. The aims in Box 4.13(a), although taken from a physiotherapy example,

Box 4.13 Aims for identified settings: physiotherapy

(a) A 20-patient acute care ward for the elderly. All patients are aged 75 years or over.

Aims:

That the student:

1. will learn how to assess, plan and carry out effective treatment for patients with multi-pathology;
2. will learn how to set realistic objectives for the elderly patient;
3. will gain an understanding of the special problems of the elderly patient group;
4. will gain experience of how to set up and carry out a home visit;
5. will gain an understanding of the different roles of all members of the multi-disciplinary team;
6. will learn to work as part of the multi-disciplinary team.

(b) Paediatric clinic. The placement is designed to allow students to gain experience in the in and out-patient treatment of children in the care and assessment centre.

Objectives specific to placement:

When you have completed this placement you should be able to:

1. explain and discuss applied anatomy and physiology and pathology of related medical, neurological and some orthopaedic conditions common in children;
2. describe respiratory assessment;
3. describe gross and fine motor development and its progression;
4. analyse gait in children;
5. discuss the psychological problems unique to children in this unit;
6. recognize and discuss the role of the physiotherapist in the assessment team and on the ward;
7. be aware of the roles of other team members;
8. have an awareness of the selection and use of aids, for example wheelchairs, corner seats, chairs, splints and shoes.

---

would be applicable across professions. It is important to set up aims which include the wider aspects of the job.

It is also important to see if student's have aims which they have set up for themselves. Knowledge of these will help you to understand what they feel about their own abilities, and what they believe they are in clinic to learn. Examples of student's own aims are shown in Boxes 4.17, (a), (b), and (c).

Box 4.14 Aims for identified settings: radiography, School of Radiography, Birmingham

---

(a) Training objectives for IVU

Care of patient

The student shall be able to:

1. describe the patient preparation necessary for IVU and state the reasons for the preparation;
2. prepare the injection tray prior to the examination;
3. explain the procedure to the patient, including length of examination;
4. suitably question the patient regarding any history of allergies;
5. state the amount and type of contrast agent used, and understand the reasons for choice of contrast agents;
6. explain the side-effects that could occur following injection of a contrast agent, and the actions required if a reaction occurs;
7. state the location and contents of emergency drug tray and resuscitation equipment.

Technique:

Students should be instructed so that they are able to undertake an IVU examination, under the supervision of a radiographer, demonstrating their ability to:

1. check the patient identification and preparation;
2. explain the procedure to the patient;
3. care for the patient in the appropriate manner;
4. assess resultant radiographs;
5. dismiss the patient with correction information on completion of the examination.

(b) Accident and emergency

Care of the patient:

The student shall be instructed to enable him/her to:

1. assess the patient's ability to cooperate with the radiographer's instructions;
2. safely manoeuvre patients with due care to the injury;
3. observe patient's clinical signs and symptoms for deterioration/change;
4. check drips for correct operation;
5. state the location and contents of emergency drugs and resuscitation equipment;
6. locate and use 'emergency buttons' as appropriate.
7. cope with patients needing special care, e.g. inebriated, aggressive;
8. identify different types of fractures.

Technique:

The student shall be encouraged to undertake techniques appropriate to the stage of training and correctly adapt the examination dependent on the patient's condition.

Box 4.14 (continued)

(c) Ward/theatre radiography

Care of the patient:

1. Assess the patient's ability to cooperate with the radiographer's instructions;
2. safely manoeuvre patients with due care to their condition;
3. observe patient's clinical signs and symptoms for deterioration/change;
4. carry out in correct manner, examination of patients under isolation conditions following guidelines issued by the control infection sister;
5. prepare self and equipment to carry out radiographic projections under asceptic conditions.

Physics equipment:

The student shall be able to:

1. apply radiation protection procedures and local rules specifically relating to mobile X-ray examinations;
2. safely manoeuvre mobile equipment within the hospital.

Technique:

The student shall be actively involved in a variety of examinations of patients on wards and in theatre.

Box 4.15 Aims for identified settings: speech and language therapy

---

(a) School for children with severe learning difficulties, Rosemary Williams, Walsall Health Authority

Approximately 80 children attend the day school, they range from 2 to 13 years. Speech therapy provision: 5 half days per week.

Role of the therapist:

To assess and provide written advice on language development, (including pre-verbal communication) and feeding difficulties. To provide planning and provision and alternative means of communication (usually with the advice of the Communication Aids link worker). To train teachers to use suitable language schemes and advise parents. To liaise with paediatric and other medical and educational staff.

Box 4.15 (continued)

Learning aims for student at the school:

I. ADMINISTRATIVE

1. Writing up case notes.
2. Making appointments with teaching staff.
3. Making appointments with parents by telephone or letter.
4. Telephoning/writing to other professionals (teachers of the visually impaired, hearing impaired, etc.).
5. Filling in statistical forms.
6. Completing inventory of equipment.
7. Extracting information from medical notes.
8. Referrals to other agencies.
9. Writing handouts for parents/teachers.
10. Time arrangement.
11. Prioritize needs of staff/children/self.
12. Learn to manage own work-load.

II. LIAISON WITH STAFF/CARERS

1. Attend meetings where appropriate.
2. Liaise with parents, teachers, ancillary staff, dinner ladies, etc. *re* language/feeding programmes.
3. Accompanying clinician on home visit.

III. PROFESSIONAL DEVELOPMENT

1. Assessment, planning treatment and implementing treatment individually or in small groups.
2. Decisions as to whether one to one or group work is appropriate and where the treatment should take place in the school setting.
3. Develop the ability to reflect on own implementation and amend plans.
4. Evaluate clinicians work.
5. Apply theory to practice.
6. Use of assessments.
7. Providing written language programmes for teaching and non-teaching staff.
8. Involvement in decisions on treatment.

(b) General hospital setting, Lorna Povey, East Birmingham Health Authority

Although there will be a wide case-load the bulk will be: voice disorders, neurological problems, laryngectomy.

General aims:

1. Give student the experience of working in a speech therapy department of a general hospital. Provide opportunity of observing different therapists working, including those not directly involved in supervision. Make student aware of the supportive role of colleagues through informal discussion, e.g. 'have you any ideas what I could do next?', 'this approach didn't work'.

Box 4.15 (continued)

2. Provide the student with opportunity to observe and describe the role of the speech therapist in hospital setting.
3. Observe a variety of patients (children and adults) with various communication problems, both on an in-patient and out-patient basis.

Specific aims:

1. To be aware of the referral system operating in the hospital and to compare it with other referral systems in the health authority.
2. Familiarize self with assessment procedures available in the department.
3. Gain knowledge of which assessment to use and why.
4. Gain experience in administration of assessments.
5. Evaluate information gained from assessments.
6. Compare informal and formal assessments and discuss their use within the hospital setting.
7. To become aware of the wider needs of the client and discuss ways these could be assessed.
8. Identify team members caring for the client.
9. To become aware of the role of the speech and language therapist as an assessor and within the team caring for the patient.

(c) General hospital outpatients, Karen Tombs, North Staffordshire Health Authority

General adult case-load – wide range of cases. Easy 'open' access to: hearing therapist; audiological services, ENT team. Opportunity for both individual and group treatments. Specific area of interest – hearing impairment in adults. Department houses Visi speech. Observation room – viewing screen into second therapy room. Opportunities for administrative procedures.

Potential for student learning:

1. Can offer patients from a wide and varied case-load to fit student needs.
2. Opportunities to observe and liaise with fellow professionals in specific areas, i.e. hearing therapist and audiological team.
3. Organizing both individual and group work as appropriate
4. Allow opportunities for administrative experience; taking 'phone calls, organizing transport, case notes, etc.
5. Prioritization of case-load.
6. Use of various assessment procedures.
7. Use of computer and Visi speech with patients.
8. Maintaining links with wards in order to obtain information relevant to the overall management of the patient. Access to patient records, etc.

Box 4.16 General aims appropriate for students in a range of settings. Adapted from Speech and Language Therapy pack, Southampton and South East Hampshire Health Authority.

Objective:

To improve the student's professional skills and knowledge other than in direct face-to-face intervention, by creating opportunities for learning in the following areas:

I.　ADMINISTRATIVE

1. Answering the telephone.
2. Writing up case notes.
3. Ordering transport and sending appointments.
4. Organizing visits to homes, schools, etc.
5. Filling in statistical information.
6. Ordering equipment.
7. Extracting/summarizing information from other professionals notes.
8. Referrals to other agencies.
9. Writing simple handouts for patients, parents and carers.

II.　LIAISON WITH STAFF/CARERS

1. Attend case conferences and staff meetings.
2. Observation of other professionals.
3. Liaise with spouses, parents, teachers, care staff, etc. in the implementation of treatment.
4. Report back to other staff on the outcomes of treatment, through discussion and written report as appropriate.

Box 4.17 Students' own goals for their clinical placements

(a) First placement

Aims for the first few weeks of a long placement:

1. To find my way round the hospital base and not get lost.
2. To talk to some hospital patients.
3. To know how I fit into the _____ Department.
4. To know what I will and will not be doing on placement.
5. To meet all the staff in the Department.
6. To learn more about how _____ fits into the hospital service as a whole.

(b) Students a few weeks into clinical experience

1. Assessment: observing _____ doing assessment and to learn how to use informal assessment myself.

Box 4.17 (continued)

---

2. To see different areas where _____ work, and learn how to interact with different people.
3. To learn about the new things I see.
4. To continue to learn about observation.
5. To continue to learn about case history taking and maybe get some practice.

(c) Students in the middle of their clinical experience and course

Student one

1. Being able to advise parents.
2. Being able to relate theory to practice.
3. Being able to break long-term goals (for the patient), into steps.
4. Being able to interpret results and draw conclusions.
5. Being confident in going on towards and dealing with new patients.

Student two

1. Take a more active role in encouraging supervisors to push me more. I feel that I'm sometimes capable of doing more, but I fail to ask to be pushed because I'm frightened of failing; if I was told to do something I would.
2. Do more administration in clinic.
3. To take initiative and not wait until somebody suggests doing something (i.e. confidence in dealing with people in higher authority).
4. To think through every case for myself and not just accept the therapist's opinion without reasoning for myself.
5. Make things more interesting for children and develop encouragement skills.

Learning contracts

Some courses encourage or even require clinical teachers to go a step further in working collaboratively with students in identifying their learning aims and needs, through learning contracts. This process is seen to be particularly valuable in the experiential learning elements of the curriculum. Tomkins and McGraw (1988) have described the learning contracts in the context of student nurses. They define contracting as 'a continuously negotiable working agreement between student and teacher, which emphasises mutality in decision making and student self determination in relation to learning outcomes'. They describe several stages in the process going from the exploration of needs, to the establishment of goals, the development of a plan, the division of responsibilities and agreement of a time frame, at the end of this there is evaluation and re-negotiation.

INFORMATION FROM THE COURSE PLACING THE STUDENT

The excellent material prepared by the receiving agencies should be matched by the information from the institution running the course. It is probably not realistic for every clinical teacher to be provided with the full course documentation, which may be very weighty and include material which will not be of particular interest to clinical teachers. However, at least one copy of the full curriculum should be housed in the receiving professional service for reference purposes. All clinical teachers could have a summary sheet of the key subject areas covered at specified stages of the course. Many clinical teachers also appreciate having a list of essential reading for students.

WELCOMING THE STUDENT TO YOUR CLINIC

The different patterns of placement across courses may require receiving agencies to think about the start of the placement for individual students in slightly different ways. The first day in an extended placement is one which is likely to have considerable impact on the student. The student starting such a placement may be away from both college and home and may feel very vulnerable. It is wise for one member of staff to plan and coordinate a fairly relaxed first day for the student, knowing that there is time ahead to cover all the many elements which need eventually to be addressed. The first day might include:

1. Set time aside to welcome – cup of coffee, warming up period!
2. Outline the opportunities available.
3. Negotiate aims and objectives for the period of the placement.
4. Discuss the students' needs, previous experiences, etc.
5. Brief introduction to resources/administration/use of phone, etc.
6. Break to meet others, have coffee/lunch, etc. It would be particularly nice for the student to meet members of staff who are not involved in their teaching, especially the recently qualified.
7. Consider just *one* patient today, student to have an observing role.
8. Set up the programme for the days ahead, with clear identification of what the student will be expected to do or bring.
9. Time to do shopping, sort out transport, etc. and make sense of what has happened during the day.

It is sad to learn that some students report that they did not feel welcomed into the placement, even expressing such feelings as; 'I felt I was in the way' or 'there wasn't time'. Busy professionals will understand how this can easily happen, but would be distressed to learn that this was the experience of students coming into their department. It is without doubt valuable to spend some time planning for the start; time taken in preparation is likely to save time later.

Box 4.18 Overall placement plan for second year student on 10-week placement: BSc Speech and Language pathology and therapeutics, Birmingham Polytechnic

The main aims of the placement are focused on patient assessment.

Week one: orientation

1. Introduce the student to the clinicians and the settings.
2. Give general organizational guidelines:
   (a) student knows starting and finishing times for clinics;
   (b) knows relevant telephone numbers;
   (c) student checks transport, timetables, etc.;
   (d) knows about emergency procedures, fire drill, health and safety;
   (e) clinical activities: student should observe one or two clients per session and discuss these with the clinician. Observations should include:
   (i) physical characteristics
   (ii) gross and fine motor behaviour,
   (iii) social interaction,
   (iv) response to general conversation,
   (v) response to specific activities in therapy.
3. Plan for some interactive task in week two.

Week two:

1. From observations, the student should describe more specific communication skills.
2. If appropriate the student should join in and spend time in play (children) or conversation with patients. The clinician should give feedback on the student's interactive skills.
3. Plan for activities student to undertake in week 3.

Week three:

1. The student may undertake a short assessment (e.g. the Edinburgh Articulation Test) under close supervision and with plenty of feedback.
2. Student should plan to analyse data collected and prepare report back by week 4.
3. Plan for the student to undertake planning of some activity by week 4, preferably related to this week's activity.

Weeks four to eight:

The student should gradually begin to develop skills in:

1. Interaction.
2. Testing.
3. Deeper understanding of communication disorders.
4. Deeper understanding of related factors, e.g. case history information, nature of the disorder and effects on family, school, work.
5. Begin to prepare case study to send tutor.

Box 4.18 (continued)

Weeks eight to ten:

If the student is ready and the case-load allows, begin to consider **the wider aspects of management**.

By week 9 the student should be preparing final reports of patients, return any case notes, complete and copy all assessments, etc. for clinic files.

When the placement is the first for a student, clinicians will wish to take particular care. When students have already done some clinical work, expectations may be different. The course or the placement may find it useful to make an overall plan for the whole of the placement period. An example is shown in Box 4.18.

When a student has already undertaken a clinical placement their expectations will be influenced by their previous experiences. It will be important to spend time exploring these, especially to understand what the student felt about the experiences.

FOLLOW-UP ACTIVITIES

1. Establish whether or not there is an information pack in your clinic/department/service. If not prepare one for your own clinical setting.
2. Devise a short questionnaire to elicit from students their own expectations about the placement.
3. Prepare a list of aims suitable for a student coming into your clinical setting, taking into account the stage of the course a student has reached and the more general aims laid down in the curriculum.
4. Draft a letter of welcome to a student appropriate to your own clinical setting.
5. Look in your own professional journals for articles on clinical teaching. What issues do they address? Make a note of each reference and list the topics which have been covered. Consider how they relate to your own work as a clinical teacher.

REFERENCES

Boyd-Webb, N. (1984) From social work practice to teaching the practice of social work. *Journal of Education for Social Work*, **20**, no. 3, 51–7.

Hanscombe, J.A. (1986) Physiotherapy – The Development of Professionalism in the Curriculum. *Physiotherapy*, **72**, 8 August, 10.

Spowart, D. (1987) Unmasking the Hidden Fears. *Therapy Weekly*, 8 October, 4.

Tomkins, C. and McGraw, M.J. (1988) The Negotiated Learning Contract, in Boud, D. (ed.) *Developing Student Autonomy in Learning*, 2nd edn, Kogan Page, London.

5

Helping students to become independent learners and professionals

INTRODUCTION

When a supportive teacher–student relationship is set up, in which the student is helped towards becoming a self-motivated, self-directed learner, then the ground is ready for the use of a number of teaching methods and the provision of opportunities which will promote the student's learning. Previous models of clinical supervision presumed that students learnt through a process of absorption. Good, well-targetted teaching procedures should be used in clinic to ensure that the student's time is productive, and that valuable staff resources are used efficiently and effectively. It is better to have less time in clinic, with good teaching, than a longer time not used purposefully.

This chapter considers some specific opportunities designed to enhance and accelerate student learning, while at the same time making the task for the teacher more concrete and specific and therefore more possible. The following methods will be considered.

- Helping the student to observe
- Teaching skills and procedures through observation and demonstration
- Helping the student to collect information
- Helping the student to fit into the team

The last two of these topics were areas identified as topics for clinical education, by the National Health Service Training Authority working party report on the Development of Supervisors of Students in Health Service Professions (1987). The working group of six who prepared this report included representatives from the majority of professions allied to medicine. It was based in North West Thames Regional Health Authority in the UK. The focus of the paper was on the clinic-based teaching of pre-registration students, as well as the establishment of a training and development programme for practitioners working with students in placement periods.

In the working party's introduction the following points are made about the attachment of student in placement, both in hospital and community settings:

1. All students in the professions represented in this project are attached to appropriate professional departments in Hospitals or Community for varying periods during their training.
2. The purpose of this attachment is to help them gain the knowledge, skills, attitudes and confidence required in making the transition from 'students in an educational establishment' to 'effective autonomous practitioner and full member of the team – with all that this implies in the change in what is expected of them by their supervisors, colleagues, patients and themselves. The educational establishments contribute much of what is needed but there is an inevitable gap between what can be achieved in an essentially academic atmosphere and what is required in the workplace with its often conflicting priorities, pressures, problems and personalities.

Some of the ideas raised in this report provide valuable starting points for the clinical teacher and will be discussed further in this chapter.

TEACHING OBSERVATIONAL SKILLS

Experienced practitioners are hardly aware of the high-level observational skills they possess. In work situations all professional groups expect students to observe what is going on; this may be directed to a number of different areas such as:

*   Patient behaviour
*   Medical conditions
*   What the clinician has done

Clinical teachers are sometimes surprised at how little students appear to have taken in, in spite of opportunities to develop observational skills in the classroom. They would also have been alerted to what they should look out for in clinic. In the place of work, however, the student might be so over-whelmed as to find it difficult to make sense of what is seen and heard. On the other hand, observing someone else doing something can be extremely 'yawn-making', especially if what the student is meant to be looking at has not been specified. There is a danger too that if observed superficially the student may think that the task is very easy and spend all the time wondering why on earth they are not allowed to get on and do it on their own. This is a natural reaction in the inexperienced health care student. Treatments which appear simple on the surface can only be carried out competently after much practice, and are often modified, while they being executed, through the clinician reflecting on what is happening and making decisions on the spot. Much of the complexity will be lost on the inexperienced/naive observer.

Clinical teachers need to make students' observational experiences as active and productive as possible, helping them not only to see what is going on at surface level, but also to be aware of the thinking activities hidden from view. This is particularly important with students at the beginning of their work experience; those further on in their course have more insight, both in skills and knowledge, on which to base their observations. It is extremely important that as clinical teachers we enable students to be effective observers, early on in their clinical experience.

Setting up the aims of observation

Periods of clinical placement which are meant to be mainly focused on observation can be difficult for both the student and the clinical teacher. It is important for clinical teachers to think about the aims of student observation, rather than letting the student have a look at anything going on. Exploration of the aims will help the clinical teacher to include a wider range of observational opportunities. The following aims are suggested:

1. To provide a clearly defined role for the student in the clinical setting.
2. To enable the student to be active in the clinical process.
3. To heighten awareness of patient behaviour.
4. To heighten awareness of clinician behaviour.
5. To learn to perform specific skills and procedures.
6. To evaluate patient behaviour.
7. To evaluate clinician behaviour.
8. To enhance understanding of specific conditions.
9. To compare patients' conditions, needs and problems.
10. To compare and contrast different clinician's approaches to management and treatment of patients.
11. To extend the understanding of patients' needs and problems, etc, by observing them in a number of different settings.
12. To help the clinician to understand the student's knowledge base and grasp of the clinical process.
13. To focus on particular aspects of the clinical process, e.g. diagnosis, counselling, treatment provisions, etc.

14. To gain an understanding of how a department operates within the total system of the hospital/clinic/school, etc.

These suggested aims remind us that in their observations, students need to focus not only on the patient, but also on the practitioner. Students will, without prompting observe and probably evaluate the work being undertaken by the practitioner. It is essential that this is focused on and explored, as a basis for the recognition of good practice. Whether it is acknowledged or not, clinicians involved in teaching students will act as powerful role models. It is particularly valuable if students are given opportunity to observe the approaches of a number of clinicians. Where students undertake placements which involve them in working with only one clinical teacher, over a considerable period of time, the influence of a single role model may not always be to the student's advantage.

It would be a good idea for the clinical teacher to sit down with the student at the beginning of the placement period to go over the aims and to draw up a list of the possible opportunities to fulfil the aims. If the observational opportunities are approached in this way the student will understand the importance of the process in their own learning, rather than seeing observation as marking time until they are allowed to get on with the job themselves. If the student is provided with clear aims for their observation they will not feel awkward but will feel part of what is going on. Clinicians may indeed find it valuable to have an extra pair of eyes, ears and hands. Focused observation will also help the student to appreciate the complexity of the clinical process even when what is being done on the surface may appear relatively simple.

You will need to consider the suggested aims of observation as listed above, in relation to the placement aims stated by the course. Taking aim 4 as an example, 'To heighten awareness of clinician behaviour', presumably a generic aim, applicable to all students. What kind of opportunities could be arranged here? The following stages are suggested:

1. Observe 'key' clinical teacher, note in particular:
    (a) interaction with patient/client;
    (b) communication –
        (i) eliciting information,
        (ii) use of questioning,
        (iii) explanations to patients,
        (iv) teaching the patient,
        (v) explaining to relatives/carers;
    (c) how does the clinical teacher relate to the team, etc?
    (d) how does the clinical teacher reach decisions on further treatment, etc?

2.   Observe another member of *same* professional field and compare/contrast the same behaviours as listed above.
3.   Observe a clinician in *another* profession, compare and contrast with your own field. Are there behaviours/skills used which could be useful in the student's own competencies? Are there other aspects which would seem inappropriate and why?

Between each of the above suggested stages, there should be a debriefing session between the student and the 'key' clinical teacher, unless the debriefing has been devolved to someone else involved in one of the stages of the observation programme.

Aims 8 and 9: 'To enhance understanding of specific conditions', and 'To compare patients' needs and problems'.

1.   Check how much the student has covered on the condition in college. If they seem vague, suggest they look at lecture notes and reading material in clinic.
2.   Has the student had access to video or audio material in college; is any available in college or clinic, to be seen in preparation? The student can arrange and do this on his/her own.
3.   Let the student observe a 'key' clinical teacher with patients/clients with specified condition. Provide guidelines for these observations (see below).
4.   Arrange a debriefing/feedback session to check on student observations. Encourage the student to further private study, if indicated. Point out any features overlooked.
5.   Let the student observe another clinical session with a 'key' clinical teacher to see if observation skills have deepened.
6.   Ask colleague if they are seeing any patients with condition X; ask if student can observe.
7.   Arrange a follow-up debriefing session for student to report back and raise any queries.
8.   If patients/clients with condition X attend for any other treatment by other professionals ask colleagues if the student may observe with them. This arrangement will help students to see patients as whole people, rather than as a specific condition. Make sure that the receiving department understands the stage the student has reached.
9.   Arrange a debriefing session.
10. If a suitable patient is under a consultant and has an appointment, see if it would be possible for the student to accompany the patient to the appointment (follow with a debriefing session).
11. Encourage the student to look back at lecture notes, which will now be more meaningful in the context of their deeper, observation-based understanding.

12. Encourage the student to record in a log book important points, especially those which they had previously not understood or misconstrued (reflection time).
13. Seek an opportunity for the student to see and recognize condition X without being alerted.

Aims for student observation are likely to vary according to the stage of the course a student has reached, as well as the particular opportunities available within a specific clinical setting. It is usually valuable to provide students with structured guidelines for carrying out observations. In the preparation of observation guidelines for the following principles are suggested:

1. Check that the physical arrangements are suitable for the student to make satisfactory observations.
2. Establish whether the student should participate or not in what is going on.
3. Decide what is to be the main focus of the observation.
4. Provide 'Bite-sized chunks' to be observed, possibly building up to the full menu! It is not necessary or helpful to try to observe a lot at first.
5. Where possible use audio- or video-recording to support the observations.
6. Get the student to make a written record of the observations they make at the time, in some ordered and manageable format.
7. If a written pro forma is to be prepared do not put too much on one sheet.
8. Focus on the here and now, especially for the beginning student.
9. Provide opportunity for discussion after the observation, so that the student gradually becomes involved in making decisions about the management of patients through analysing and evaluating what has taken place.
10. Encourage the student to be aware of the practitioner's thinking throughout the clinical process.
11. Don't give the student too much information about a patient, as this may restrict their own thinking.
12. Arrange opportunities for observation both in your own department and with the rest of the multiprofessional team.
13. With experience, students may be able to devise their own observation schedules.

Many teachers in both the classroom and the clinic, have a tendency to make tasks too complex for students. This may be particularly true in setting up observation guidelines. Without guidance students often feel that they have to observe everything. It is very rare that a task is made too simple for the learner; simple tasks can serve to make students feel good, knowing that they can cope, especially early on in their clinical experience. It does not harm the experienced clinician when students say to their peers that something was 'dead simple' or 'fancy asking me to do that!'

The post-observation discussion provides the opportunity to discover, either overtly or covertly, just how deep an understanding the student really has. Tasks set at too high a level may result in the student not feeling able to cope and being a failure. It may in fact prevent them from coping in areas which are in fact well within their competence. Clinical teachers will quickly become aware of the level at which students are able to function and can, if necessary, stretch them further during discussions following an observation and increase the difficulty of the observational task.

Clinical teachers sometimes have a tendency to tell students too much about the patients they are going to observe. This deprives the student of the opportunity of carrying out some of the problem-solving activities which the clinician has already undertaken. Students should be provided with information which is essential for the patient's physical and emotional well-being, as well as with the kind of information which all clinicians would be provided with when first seeing a new case. Holding back additional information which is known to the clinician can provide excellent learning opportunities for the student. It also helps them to feel that they can make a real contribution and that the clinical teacher's decisions are not immutable and new ideas can be suggested. This approach may also begin to lay down the message that, on qualification, clinicians do not possess all the answers.

I first came across well-directed observational guidelines in the speech and language therapy field. The clinical teacher presumed that all clinical teachers used similar guidelines. My own experience and enquiries suggest that they are used only rarely. Discussion with clinical teachers from other fields shows that they are only occasionally used. Although the two following examples are from speech and language therapy they are simple enough to be accessible to all professional groups and could therefore be understood by inexperienced students. They were designed for second year students undertaking their first period of work experience. The setting was a community clinic for children with developmental, speech and language problems. The guidelines for observing Lynne found in Box 5.1a, is a masterpiece of simplicity. Note how little information is provided. Note how Question 2, although not asking the student what the presenting problems are (which could make the student anxious) does, nevertheless, require that the student has observed the condition to some extent, in order that an appropriate assessment tool may be selected. See how the clinical teacher encourages the student to get inside the clinician's head, as well as to feel good by telling the clinician what she 'should be thinking'. Question 1 is low key and unthreatening; not asking students to 'describe the presenting speech' but only asking them to do as much as they can manage. What a confidence builder this is. The clinical teacher will easily be able to evaluate how much the student has taken in about the presenting

Box 5.1 Observation guideline: speech and language therapy student, early on in clinical experience, Val Dinning, Walsall Health Authority

---

(a) Observation of Lynne, 2 years old:

I have only just begun seeing this little girl for a session of regular therapy.

1. Comment as you can on her presenting speech.
2. What assessment should I be thinking of making?

(b) Observation of Paul, 6 years:

This is a review appointment for Paul; he has not been seen for 6 months. He was first seen in clinic 18 months ago with delayed phonological development. There has been good progress but certain phonemes are not established.

1. Which are the phonemes?
2. Which aspects of his phonological system are still unstable?
3. I am to make a decision as to whether to treat again now or leave. What are some of the considerations which might be going through my head?

---

problems, thus leading to either more specific direction in the future or work which will lead the student on to more complex understandings.

The second example, for Paul (Box. 5.1b), again illustrates the brevity of information provided. The first part requires the students to focus quite specifically on the speech of the child, without asking them to do too much. In Question 3, again the clinical teacher tries to encourage the students to be aware that thinking is an essential part of practice. The clinician does not, however, ask for all the considerations but just some of them. Again, this kind of approach provides opportunity for the students to respond at various levels but not to fail. One hopes that the answer to question 3 would not be 'I don't know!'

The principles illustrated in these observational guidelines can be applied to students in all health care groups. Clinicians from all fields who have tried using observation guidelines with students have found them very productive both as teaching and learning devices. Boxes 5.2 to 5.7 give examples from a number of different fields.

In the context of achieving the specific aim of enhancing understanding about a specific condition, it would be useful to have a prepared guideline for use by students in clinical session, in which a number patients, with generally the same condition, are attending for assessment or routine follow-up. Once prepared, this type of guideline (e.g. Box 5.2c), can

Box 5.2 Observation guideline: chiropody/podiatry student

(a) Observation guide for second-year student: Mr Smith

Mr Smith has been rheumatoid for 10 years. He has begun complaining of his feet hurting when he walks.

1. Observe the quality and range of joint motion within the mid-tarsal, sub-talar and metatarso-phalangeal joints.
2. Do the joints feel normal?
      is the range of motion excessive, normal or limited?
      is the quality of motion good?
      is the movement roughened, notchy or smooth?
3. Suggest some possible causes for your findings.

(b) John Smith

John Smith is 14 years old. He is 6 foot 6 inches tall and has flat fleet.

Please observe John's posture and gait as I get him to walk up and down the clinic, pay particular attention to:

- the level of his shoulders;
- the arm swing;
- the position of the patellae;
- the position of the back of the heel.

Record the observation on the assessment sheet. Are there any other observations you have made. Looking at the observations can you see any that are abnormal. If so what should the ideal/normal observation be. By looking at these results please suggest a possible diagnosis that could be arrived at.

(c) These patients have been seen by the foot care assistant and need their yearly assessment

1. Note how the patients bend to remove their shoes, socks, etc.
2. Have they cut their toe nails? Have they been successful in this?
3. Note the colour of the skin.
4. Note the temperature of the skin, e.g. cold to touch.
5. Are the shoes a good fit? Measure the feet (a) at rest (b) standing. If you think the shoes are not the correct size, draw round the shoe, then draw round the foot. Examine the difference.

---

be photocopied and will be readily available to give to students, thus saving the clinical teacher's time. Before you have a lot of copies done, be sure to ask some students on their value. Better still, hold the information on computer so that it can be easily updated and printed out when required.

The guideline in Box 5.2c is good because it also gives the student a specific but simple task to undertake (draw round the shoe, then draw round the foot). Point 3 in Box 5.2a, 'Suggest some possible causes for your findings', is

Box 5.3 Observation guideline: dietetics student

(a) Mr Strong

Mr Strong is an amateur weight lifter who has been told that he must lose weight following appendicectomy. Coronary heart disease runs in the family and this appears to be the prime motivation for the medical team to prescribe weight reduction.

I know very little about weightlifting and we have not had time to prepare. We cannot weigh on our scales. He says he weighs 24 stone.

1. What kind of thoughts do you think are going through my mind?
2. As far as you know do you think we are justified in asking this patient to lose a lot of weight?
3. Are there any signs as to whether or not he wants to lose weight;
4. Has he had any nutritional education from his coach?
5. Is he prepared to weigh himself and tell us the results?

(b) Mrs Brown

Mrs Brown is a pregnant woman who has been shown to have diabetes, related to pregnancy. The doctor will start her on twice daily injections and has referred her to us for dietary education. This is her first appointment. In your observations consider the following:

1. The methods I use to keep my initial contact simple and effective, for this woman, who is under a lot of pressure.
2. How she views her current eating habits.
3. How willing she is to make changes.
4. What are the time constraints on the dietary education programme?
5. How do you think I can motivate her to continue her dietary education?

(c) Mr Payne

Mr Payne is a patient who requires long-term nutritional support. He is undergoing treatment for leukaemia. He is underweight and has a poor appetite. He is presently at home being treated as an out-patient. Observe me interviewing Mr P. and consider the following questions.

1. What is your initial impression of Mr P.?
2. How will we find out about Mr P's present attitude to food?
3. Who else might be involved in supporting Mr P. to check his diet?
4. What data do you think could be used to monitor Mr P's. progress? Would it be readily available?

Box 5.4 Observation guideline: occupational therapy student

(a) Mrs A.

Mrs A is 75 years old, and has had a right CVA, resulting in a left hemiplegia. We are still assessing her functional capabilities particularly with regard to perceptual difficulties. We are going to do a simple kitchen assessment and get her to self-propel from corridor to kitchen:

1. Observe her mobility in a wheelchair:
   (a) what problems might she have which indicate a perceptual problem?
   (b) how did the therapist help her to be aware of these?
2. Observe Mrs A. making a hot drink:
   (a) what were her specific problems with this?
   (b) can you outline which perceptual deficits may be evident?
   (c) how might you assess this further?
   (d) what did the OT do/say to overcome this?

(b) Miss E.

Miss E. is 74 years old; she had a left hemiplegia six months ago.

1. Observe her posture sitting in a chair. How might this be improved?
2. Observe how she takes off her blouse. What problems does she have?
3. Observe how she transfers from chair to bed. Did she have any problems and how safe was she?

(c) Mrs Jones. Also suitable for physiotherapy student

Mrs Jones is 84 and lives on her own in a terraced house. She returned home from the general hospital 3 days ago following internal fixation of her fractured neck of femur, which she sustained after a fall downstairs 6 weeks ago.

We are visiting her for the first time today since her discharge:

1. Start observing when we reach the house:
   (a) how long does she take to answer the door?
   (b) note any walking aids, is she using them correctly?
2. During discussion with her:
   (a) how does she appear to be coping?
   (b) is she anxious/confident/confused?
3. What does she feel are her major concerns/difficulties?
4. What would you think are her major difficulties?
5. Observe her functional activity. Can she manage important transfers independently? e.g. stairs, sit-to-stand and vice versa.
6. Can she manage activities of daily living independently? e.g. washing, dressing, preparing a meal.
7. Can you suggest any aids which might help her perform these activities more easily? e.g. toilet raise, chair raise, kitchen aids.

a very good way to try to elicit the information in an unthreatening way. The debriefing session will help to clarify the student's level of understanding. Examples (a) and (b) are both helpful in structuring exactly what the student has to look out for, i.e. the three points for assessing the feelings of the joints and the features to look at in observing John's posture and gait. Initially do not make the observational instructions too vague; give the student structured pointers, until you feel confident that they will routinely observe in a structured way.

Box 5.3a is also good in encouraging the student to get inside the clinician's head. Question 3 requires that the student listens very carefully to what the patient says, a skill which needs to be established early on in the developing health professional. In 5.3b. Question 1 is particularly valuable in encouraging the student to attend to the clinician's behaviour, this is an area that perhaps we don't pay enough attention to in observations. Question 5 'How do you think I can motivate her to continue her dietary education', may be too complex for the inexperienced observer. Perhaps this kind of question could be raised in the debriefing session, rather than written down in the guideline. It may be that the student will spend too much time thinking about it when he/she should be concentrating on observing what is going on.

In Box 5.4b, would it be sufficient to observe the patient's posture, especially for the inexperienced student (Question 1). In the debriefing session it will probably become evident whether the student can handle suggestions for improvement. It is important to remember that domiciliary work with patients also requires structured observational guidelines. Visiting a patient's home may be particularly distracting for the student and they may easily miss a number of important points. It is clearly important for students to accompany clinicians on home visits, and to get as much out of them as possible.

Box 5.5a illustrates well how a student can be involved in what is going on; 'Please help me by recording the measurements accurately and clearly'. Question 5 is important in helping the student to understand the clinicians decision-making processes. The schedule in Box 5.5a is similar to that in 2, in that it can be used on similar clinical occasions. Box 5.5a achieves a nice balance between clinical accuracy and attending to the needs and feelings of the patients.

If the student is involved in a situation where a number of patients/clients are present at one time, for example, in a school setting, in a CDC, in treatment of a group of patients, in a day centre, etc., it is a good idea to get the student to select one patient for the focus of their observation, unless they are learning to observe the functioning of the group. An example is shown in Box 5.5b. This also includes the question 'How does he/she make contact with the other children in the group?', clearly an important question where the clinical concern encompasses the patient/client in a social context, such as children with special needs, psychiatric work, and patients with communication disorders.

Box 5.5 Observation guideline: orthoptics student

(a) Synoptophore tests

This morning I will be carrying out synoptophore tests, in nine positions of gaze, with several patients. I want you to observe the following:

1. How I explain the test to the patient.
2. How I set the patient correctly and comfortably for the test.
3. Please help me by recording the measurements accurately and clearly.
4. Do you have any ideas how these measurements relate to the conditions found in the patients?
5. Why do you think I decided it was necessary to carry out this test with each of the patients concerned.

(b) Child development

You will be spending the morning in the play area of the child development centre. I want you to select one child in particular. Make the following observations:

1. What is his/her physical appearance like?
2. What in particular do you notice about his/her eyes?
3. How does he/she make contact with the other children in the group?
4. Which toys does he/she choose to play with? Have you any ideas why this might be?
5. How does he/she relate to the nursery nurses?

It is clearly a good idea to help a student to get more out of a visit to theatre by structuring their observation (Box 5.6a). It is especially important to structure observation when the situation is so unfamiliar and frightening that it has the potential to overwhelm the student and become wasted as a learning experience. Perhaps Question 6, which follows on from the observation should be asked in the follow-up session. The student will no doubt have plenty to think about during the operation. I like Question 1 in Box 5.6b, 'What words could you use to describe her behaviour?' This seems to signal to the student that lay terms are acceptable and that what is important is the observation, and not necesssarily having the correct terms. Including the student by getting him/her to ask the patient about their problem is a good idea. Box 5.6c is also a good example of grading the student's involvement in doing things with patients (Can you take off his socks? What did you notice about the feel of his legs?)

Box 5.7a is another example of a way to direct the student's observation in an area where there is a lot to observe, and the student may not know how to tackle it. The guidance in Box 5.7d, although directed to James, includes

Box 5.6 Observation guideline: physiotherapy student

(a) Physiotherapy student visiting neurosurgery theatre, patient synopsis
Young woman with one year history with balance (?problems) and RT facial
weakness. The CT scan shows a large benign cerebellar tumour.

1. What position was the patient in during the operation?
2. How did the surgeon open the skull?
3. How large was the tumour and what was the colour of it?
4. Try and describe how it differed from the surrounding brain tissue.
5. What sort of things did the surgeon point out to you?
6. Try and think of some of the considerations I will be making when I
   see this lady post-op tomorrow. i.e. what sort of things could I look
   at when I assess her?.

(b) Physiotherapy in psychiatry
A 23-year-old woman has knee pain, and walks on both toes. We have
success during treatment but she has difficulty in between treatment.

1. What words could you use to describe her behaviour?
2. After watching me work with the patient:
   (a) what do you see as her main problems?
   (b) ask the patient what she sees as her main problems.
3. Can you think of any other ways to help her maintain her exercises
   at home?
4. For what reasons do you think she finds this difficult?

(c) Cerebral palsy

Robert is 3 years old and has cerebral palsy. He has a spastic right side
and is coming in for a swim.

1. When he arrives, watch how he sits in his pushchair and compare this
   with the way he sits on his mother's lap.
2. Watch how his mother takes off his jumper.
3. Can you take off his socks? What did you notice about the feel of his
   legs?
4. Why do you think swimmning might help him?

---

principles of observation of feeding which could be more widely applied.
When preparing observation guidelines you may find that you can gradually
develop some which can be used with a number of different patients. These
will provide a very valuable resource and be timesaving. In debriefing
sessions you can make sure that you follow up points that have particular
importance for individual patients. You can also easily delete a point from
a general guideline which you feel a student is not ready to cope with.

Box 5.7 Observation guideline: speech and language therapy student

---

(a) Motor neurone disease case

Female, 58 years

1. How easy/difficult was communication between 'patient' and therapist? What strategies do they both use to aid communication?
2. Observe the patient's swallowing mechanism. Is there anything unusual about it, such as posture, initiation, speed etc.?

(b) Developmental delay, venue: child development centre:

Female, 12 months

Observe Emma's responses to other children.
Comment on:

1. her response to other's vocalization;
2. any physical contact attempted;
3. any interest in the activities of others.

(c) Cerebral vascular accident

Male, 65 years

Mr H. had a CVA 6 weeks ago; he is having regular therapy.

1. What physical effects has the CVA had?
2. What comprehension does he appear to have?
3. How does he communicate?
4. What difficulties does he have with speaking?

(d) Severe learning difficulties

James is severely mentally and physically disabled; he is 28 years old. He has spent the last 20 years in hospital. He is following a feeding programme which has been running for 2 months.
The aims decided on with John's key worker are to assist John to:

    (a) feed himself with a spoon;
    (b) become more independent.

Method:

1. Helper has hand over John's as he holds the spoon.
2. Assists loading the spoon.
3. Prompts direction of the spoon.
4. Encourages the correct direction of the spoon.

Observation:

1. **Sitting.** Is John well aligned in the chair?
2. **Head position.** Is it back/forward/normal?
3. **Position of helper.** Opposite/behind?
4. **Utensils.** Are they appropriate? Are they adapted specially?

Can you comment on points 3 and 4 of the methods and decide if, in your opinion, the process is agreeable to John. Comment on the observed relationships with the helper.

Box 5.7 (continued)

(e) Voice problem

Mrs A. is attending her first speech therapy appointment. She has been referred by an ENT consultant. She has a 6-month history of a voice problem. Indirect laryngoscopy shows the cords to be red and thickened.

1. What are your immediate impressions of Mrs A.'s voice?
2. Comment on her posture and presentation of self.
3. What sort of questions might I want to ask Mrs A. about her voice?
4. What aspects of Mrs A.'s speech/voice should I think about assessing?

Box 5.8 Observation guideline: feeding of a cerebral palsied child

---

Date　　　　　　　　　Name of child
Setting　　　　　　　　Age

FACTORS TO OBSERVE IN DRINKING AND FEEDING

1. Is it dependent or independent feeding?
2. If dependent, who is involved?
3. Are any special appliances used to help feeding? If so what are they? What purpose are they serving?
4. What proportion of food is actually swallowed?
5. Does food actually stay in the mouth?
6. If food exudes from the mouth is this: hardly at all/a little/a lot?
7. What are the possible reasons for loss of food from the mouth? Tongue thrust? Lolling tongue? Poor lip seal? Other reasons?
8. Position of head in swallowing?
9. Spontaneous or assisted swallow? Note the type of food in relation to ability to swallow.
10. Observe the length of chewing time on bolus.
11. Estimate the overall length of feeding time.

Questions 3 and 4 in Box 5.7e are further examples of helping the student to think like a clinician.

Most of the examples are well targetted at the specified professional group. However, some of the examples could well be used across professions and could be useful when students from another profession observe in your department. For example the observation of James, aged 28 years, who is severely physically handicapped (see Box 5.7d) could be used by students from physiotherapy, occupational therapy and speech and language therapy.

Box 5.9 Time sampled observation of child in classroom, to be carried out by student

---

Attending to the teacher

Student observes David in the classroom setting. He is to be observed in particular to record his ability to attend to the teacher.

Attending means **looking at the teacher** when the teacher is:

(a) talking to the class;
(b) demonstrating an activity to the class;
(c) talking to David;
(d) demonstrating an activity to David.

Observation is to be recorded at points of time, as indicated below.

TIME	IS TEACHER REQUIRING ATTENTION?	IS DAVID LOOKING AT THE TEACHER?
9.00		
9.05		
9.10		
9.15		
9.20		
9.25		
9.30		
9.35		
9.40		

Time would cover one lesson period

As students become more experienced, the observational guidelines can become more complex, with regard to the amount and difficulty of the material the student is required to observe and the level of involvement in what is happening. Box 5.8 is an example of a more complex observation guideline, on the feeding of a cerebral palsied child; again it could be useful for more than one professional group.

Some of the observational guidelines may involve time sampling, thus preparing the student for the kind of observation procedures which may be used as a research as well as a clinical tool. An example using time sampling is shown in Box 5.9.

Through carefully graded observation the student can gradually become involved in what is being done with the patient. The student and clinician slowly and almost imperceptibly can reach a stage in which they are sharing the undertaking of the treatment of the patient, as well as sharing the decisions which need to be made. Students find this approach reassuring and supportive. The clinical teacher can carefully monitor how the student is managing and gradually assign more of the treatment and responsibility to them.

There are a number of different subjects which would be suitable for student observation. Apart from the suggestions which follow, you will have other ideas from knowledge of your own field.

1. The individual treatment of patients.
2. Group treatment: groups as a whole, one patient within a group.
3. Different contexts, e.g. the ward; the day unit; the community clinic; child assessment unit; special educational setting.
4. A number of different patients with the same condition/lesion/disorder to compare and contrast.
5. One patient in different settings, for example how does the hemiplegic patient cope in: the ward; in physiotherapy, in occupational therapy; in speech and language therapy; at home.
6. The functioning of the team.
7. How clinical sessions operate.
8. How does a child interact in different settings: at home; in school; in the special unit; with his peers; with his parents.
9. How does a special unit operate, e.g. geriatric unit; mental handicap unit; the child development centre, etc.
10. Diagnostic procedures, X-rays, screening procedures, etc.

A group of clinical teachers in chiropody/podiatry drew up the following list of topics as being suitable subjects for student observation:

- Circulation
- Nail care
- Correlation of wear on footwear to foot
- Assessment of gait – child and adult
- Range of assessment procedures
- Domiciliary visits
- Diabetic ulcers and other lesions
- Procedures for strapping and padding
- Nail deformities
- Hemiplegia and footwear
- Comparing and contrasting patients with the same condition

Once you get into the habit of preparing observation guidelines you will find that you can prepare them very quickly. The written record of completed observations will provide excellent material for the student's log book. Sometimes students make original observations which contribute to or even alter the management of the case.

TEACHING CLINICAL PROCEDURES

It is only a short step from structured observations to teaching a student to carry out a specific procedure, through observation and demonstration. The example in Box 5.8 which is specifically designed to get the student to observe a severely physically handicapped child feeding, at the same time begins to prepare the student for undertaking working with the child.

When an actual assessment instrument, diagnostic investigation, treatment procedure or technical skill is to be taught it is important that the task is broken down into carefully graded steps. Crago and Pickering (1987), quote the schedule devised by Rassi (1978), from the clinical teaching of audiology students. An examination of these principles, listed below (with some additions) shows that the principles of this schedule could readily be applied to all fields. The stages of teaching a procedure are as follows:

1. **Detailed explanation** with accompanying demonstration of every action from the beginning to the end of the procedure.
2. **General explanation** with some accompanying demonstration of every action from the beginning to the end of the procedure.
3. **Suggestions or corrections** while student is performing the task.
4. **Pre-structuring of task beforehand**, with special reminders about safety, with no explanation while the student is performing.
5. **Instruction on what task is to be performed** and its underlying rationale, but no explanation of how to do it before, during or after the performance, unless there is danger to the patient or the student.
6. **Review with student beforehand** tasks to be performed, with the student making all the decisions, the clinical teacher only making suggestions where necessary.
7. **Review of tasks after their completion**.
8. **Student makes all the decisions, performs all the tasks; Supervisor monitors; suggests only when deemed necessary**.

Examples of the steps in teaching a procedure can be found in Boxes 5.10–5.13. The first one (5.10), prepared by an occupational therapist working in the community, is of a general nature, and would be useful in all fields, while the others relate to the specific nature of the clinical work undertaken. The example in Box 5.13 illustrates teaching a student to use an assessment

Box 5.10 A prescriptive teaching guide for accessing information. Pauline Sweeting, Occupational Therapist

---

Performing a computer search to establish whether or not the person is known to the social services department, and to establish the status of the case.

Teaching guidelines:

1. Clinical teacher runs through procedure on own to make sure of own competence and to highlight any particular pitfalls in the procedure.
2. With the student present, who has a good view of the screen, demonstrate and talk through the procedure. Student to make own notes for future reference. Demonstration to focus only on the task in hand and not to digress.
3. Student to carry out computer search using own notes as guidelines and asking questions if necessary. Teacher to prompt if student stuck or has gone badly wrong. Repeat until the student can do on own only with recourse to own notes.
4. Provide opportunities soon afterwards for student to do search on own. Point out and introduce to members of the clerical team who can be called on if in difficulty.

---

tool for language in a post-stroke adult. It includes consideration of the criteria for use of the procedure. This is an important stage on from the actual proficiency of the use of a procedure as it helps students to be able to select appropriate procedures on their own in the future. The evaluative aspect needs to be incorporated into learning about all procedures.

Additional questions for the clinical teacher to ask the student following the use of a diagnostic or evaluation procedure would be:

1. Do you think the results of your assessment were reliable, and if not why not?
2. How are you going to use the information gained from your assessment in the management of the patient?
3. What further assessments/procedures should be carried out?
4. Who should be informed of the assessment findings and how should this be done?
5. Are there any ethical considerations relating to the procedure?
6. What are the safety concerns related to the procedure?

With some assessment tools it will be necessary to discuss with the student such matters as; the effect of patient cooperation on the results, test validity and standards scores.

Box 5.11 Teaching a student to make a special pad. Anne Locke, Chiropodist, Southampton

1. **Clinical teacher** explains exactly what is going to be taught and why this particular superimposed crescent pad is being used. Explains the materials necessary, etc.
2. Makes the pad at normal speed.
3. Makes the pad slowly, breaking the method down into separate components. Uses verbal explanation as proceeds.
4. Gives student 'crib card' and allows student to read card and ask any questions.
5. **Student** makes pad following tutor's verbal instructions.
6. Tutor makes the pad following instructions given by **the student** using the 'crib card'.
7. Student makes pad on own following 'crib card' as necessary.
8. Student makes pad on own gradually, with no directions from teacher or 'crib card'.

The crib card

Use of the superimposed crescent pad. Infected corn or inflamed area over interphalangeal joint on 2nd, 3rd or 4th toes, usually in hammer or flexed position.

Materials:
5 mm or 7 mm semi-compressed wool felt (according to depth being filled). Appropriate medication and gauze. Tubular gauze, size 12. Chirofix.

Method:

1. Choose thickness of felt required to fill the gap between dorsum of foot and top of lesion.
2. Cut crescent pad with 'arms' just long enough to meet round the lesion, using top third of pad.
3. Cut piece of felt the same length and shape as before, but this time with slight 'V' at top end to fit snugly up to the toe.
4. Stick crescent to filler pad with top end of crescent free.
5. Trim round the whole pad reducing it to nothing at the distal edge, making it smooth with no ridges.
6. Remove a small amount of adhesive where the pads fit round the lesion. (Feathering).
7. Prepare skin and apply the dressing. Firmly stick pad in place, covering with tubular gauze and securing with Chirofix.
8. Give the patient instructions on the care of the pad.

Box 5.12 Guidelines for applying an ice pack in physiotherapy

Student has already covered the theory underlying the use of ice in college and has made and applied an ice pack on a student model.

These guidelines are issued when the student observes the clinician applying an ice pack to a patient, prior to the student doing it to a patient.

1. Make the patient comfortable, expose the area to be treated.
2. Examine the skin for temperature, odour, intactness.
3. Put plastic sheet under patients limb, put towel on top of plastic sheet.
4. Apply oil to area to be treated. Do not forget posterior aspects, if ice is going to be in contact.
5. Apply ice pack. Secure with towel and plastic. Leave for 15 minutes.
6. Remove icepack. Dry and wash oil off. Remove towel and plastic sheet.
7. Inspect skin for temperature and erythema.

Box 5.13 Stages in teaching the administration and selection of an aphasia assessment. Nanette Maver, Speech and Language Therapist, Swindon.

1. Preparation – student takes away the complete test, to read, study and familiarize (will no doubt have already been introduced in college; clinical teacher will check previous experience).
2. Clinical teacher and student meet to discuss the best procedure, student brings queries.
3. Clinical teacher administers test to patient, student watches with guidance for particular points to observe.
4. Student practices administration of test with peers, clinicians, etc.
5. Clinical teacher again administers test to patient, student records responses of patient on appropriate forms.
6. Clinician discusses and evaluates patient responses.
7. Student writes up results on appropriate forms/sheets/case notes.
8. Student administers test to patient *and* records responses.
9. Clinical teacher provides opportunity for student to test other patients when possible.
10. Student and clinical teacher discuss the criteria to be used in selecting the test for particular patients.
11. Student and clinical teacher discuss alternative assessments and their relative merits.

All these ideas have much greater learning value when discussd and related to a known case, rather than being addressed only in the sterile context of the classroom. Reviewing the procedures undertaken by the student is usually best done through discussion immediately after working with a patient, if this is possible. In some instances the student may need to be given time to analyse complex material in more depth and to reflect on what has happened, before reaching conclusions, both in relation to the patient's needs and in relation to how the student carried out the task or procedure. A busy clinical session is not readily geared to this; the clinical teacher needs to ensure that 'thinking space' is created for the student. Fish *et al.* (1990) stress the importance of reflection not only after but also during pratice. In order to achieve time to think during the process clinicians and students need to feel 'comfortable' with what they are doing. If students are made to carry out procedures with which they are not adequately prepared, they will not be able to think through them, because their anxiety will interfere with their thinking. These points will be discussed further in Chapter 7.

Clinical teachers in some fields report that lecturers in some colleges do not like students to be provided with 'crib sheets' or guidelines for carrying out procedures, such as suggested in Box 5.11. This view is difficult to understand. Certainly one would not wish students to be confused by different instructions, but students do need to learn that there may be slightly different, but acceptable ways of doing things. Such a directive from a course seems to have two unfortunate hidden messages; (i) the way which is prescribed by college staff is the only way and (ii) that the status of what is taught in college overrides the status of what is taught in clinic. The use of a crib sheet may in fact help the student to be less anxious with the procedure and therefore enable them to concentrate more on what is happening to the patient. Where questions on safety are involved the judgement of the clinical teacher supervising the student at the time, who is also responsible for the patients, must take precedence over any instructions received by the student from other sources.

HELPING STUDENTS TO COLLECT INFORMATION

Some areas which are central to competence and professional effectiveness cannot be learnt purely through observation, demonstration and practice. The areas are more subtle and require that clinical teachers consider what can be done to enable these competences to be developed. The two areas identified by the National Health Service Training Authority (NHSTA) are:

- Helping the student to collect information
- Helping the student to fit into the team

The NHSTA working party (1987) suggested that the following areas needed to be considered in helping students to collect information:

1. Referral notes;
2. X-rays;
3. Case history;
4. Patient reports;
5. Physical examination;
6. Observations.

It may be helpful to break down the components into other categories. The above list suggests that all information is patient related, it may however need to be wider than this. The following six headings are suggested.

1. **Practical**
   (a) Straightforward non-controversial factual material can be provided in a written form, such as is prepared by the health authority or by the service or department in a student information pack; see Chapter 4.
   (b) A student induction session will help to clarify points and provide additional information.
   (c) Early on in the student's clinical experience attempts should be made to create an open, welcoming atmosphere in which students feel they can seek information.
   (d) Introduce ancillary/support staff to the student as they may be of importance in information gathering.
2. **Administration**
   (a) It may be best to introduce students to various administrative procedures through the needs of an individual case. This will help to provide a framework to help the student remember the procedure, for example, how to access patient data, order transport, etc. Such information served out cold is difficult to remember.
3. **Patient information**
   (a) Files: where are they? how are they accessed? when should a student write in/add to them? what has to be done with them after use?
   Patient information needs to be as available to students as to professionals.
   (b) A student's first attempt at obtaining information from a professional colleague can be eased by the cooperation of other staff, for example arranging for the student to speak to an approachable 'ward sister', school head, consultant, etc. for the first occasion that the student has to gather information from another person in the health, education or social service team.

4. **Academic information**
   (a) Introducing the student to library facilities; postgraduate, general and departmental. Students from an institution of higher education can be given a letter of introduction to an institutional library, such as that of a university or polytechnic, in the locality of the placement. This will be particularly important for students on long placements away from their college base.
   (b) List of and access to journals subscribed to by members of staff.
   (c) Introduction to personnel who may have particular interests, e.g. departmental staff engaged in projects, other staff in the locality with special interests/expertise.
   (d) Inviting student to professional meetings, study days, etc.
5. **State and voluntary support schemes**
   (a) It is important that students are made aware of the state and voluntary institutions which may be available to support specific client groups.
   (b) The student should be familiar with the literature which is available to patients, from these organizations.
   (c) Lists of organizations should be held by the service. The particular profession will hold contact names and addresses of organizations related to client groups with which the department works.
   (d) Keeping an eye on the press is helpful in identifying what local groups are doing, a student may be interested in keeping an eye on the press for the department, during the period of the placement.
   (e) It may be possible to arrange for the student to attend patient support group meetings, a valuable opportunity in helping to achieve a holistic view of patients/clients.
6. **Personal**
   (a) Students need access to information about themselves and their progress. This can be provided by the clinical teacher and college tutor through feedback. (This will be addressed more fully in Chapter 7).
   (b) Clinicians need time to provide feedback to students. It is highly unlikely that a full case-load can be maintained by the clinical teacher when student teaching/supervision is added to the work-load.

The NHSTA working party suggested five points which need to be considerd when information has been collected:

1. **Ordering and analysis of information**. Do students know what to extract out of the ward notes, or from the hospital notes where a patient was seen 10 years ago. Can they then analyse the information into something meaningful for their own needs?

2. **Exercising clinical judgment** in establishing goals of therapy and developing alternative strategies.

3. **Selecting the strategy likely to be the most successful within the constraints of the situation**. Students should not always be directed in what to do in the treatment of a case. They need the opportunity to establish their own goals, both long and short term, for the patient, as well as to develop stragtegies/procedures/treatments to help the patient reach these goals.

4. **Action**. Is the management of the case to be undertaken by oneself or others. Can the student reach this decision? Can the student enlist the cooperation of others in implementation?

5. **Control**. Is the student aware of the need to continue to observe and evaluate the outcomes of intervention against what has been expected?

The clinical teacher needs to be mindful of all these points and to ensure that the student has had the opportunity to develop competence in all these areas.

HELPING THE STUDENT TO FIT INTO THE TEAM

The teams in health, in education and in social services are complex ones. Some health care workers are involved in case work which requires relationships with staff in all three services. This is a demanding aspect of the work for the student to enter into. It is not easy for students to become good team members in practice, if they hear about the ideal of team work only in the classroom, and do not encounter the reality of it in their work experience. Professionals act as powerful role models in team work, so clinical teachers need to ensure that students have opportunities to experience team work both through observing it in practice and in having the opportunity gradually to become part of a team.

Clinical teachers will recognize that students need to be allowed to 'get their feet wet' in those parts of the job that are difficult and less easily controlled by the clinical teacher. Working in the team falls into this category. The following ideas have been generated from discussion across professional groups and are offered as a starting point in relation to helping students to fit into teams:

1. **Ensure that the student has ample opportunity to fit into 'the home' professional team**. This might initially be done informally, but should also include attendance at staff meetings, journal clubs, special interest groups, training days, seminars, etc. Observing other clinicians working, who may not be involved in teaching the student. Ability to fit into the 'home team' needs to be demonstrated before the student is expected to become a team member with others outside the professional group.

2. **Who is the team?** Explore the team make-up relevant to particular client groups, management and administration, etc. This would be a good topic for a student to address in a new placement.

3. **Written information.** The departmental profile provided for the student may include names and contact numbers of the home team. Where the profession has regular interface with a range of team members it could be of value to provide a list of key personnel. This will reduce some of the anxiety for the student in remembering people's names on introduction.

4. **Meeting team members informally.** Casual meetings over coffee, in the corridor or staff room can help others to recognize the new student, while the student can gradually be introduced to team members in a situation which does not make any professional demands.

5. **Observing others.** Arrange for the student to spend some time observing the work of other team members. This will increase the student's understanding of that professional role and facilitate effective liaison. It will help the student to see that all team members have equal contributions to case management. It may be particularly useful for the student to note areas of overlap in team work, these may be areas for good cooperation or alternatively areas of potential conflict.

6. **Prompts for interaction.** With inexperienced students it may be necessary to give them reminders to refer/participate with, involve/inform other team members. This may be necessary in particular in relation to parents, relatives, carers, etc. Remember to build in opportunities for liaison with voluntary and charitable organizations. The student should gradually become independent in participating and maintaining interaction with the team.

7. **Alert team members.** It may help to remind other team members that a new student has joined the department. A pro forma memo might be useful in circulating the name. Where possible let team members know the level of participation to expect from the student. Contact the professionals involved, to prepare the ground and goodwill. Team members will often provide useful feedback to the clinical teacher on how a student managed.

8. **More formal meetings with team members.** Encourage the student to see other team members to gather information or discuss management of specific cases. The clinical teacher can help to build the student's confidence by pre-structuring the interview, possibly requiring the student to draw up the aims for the planned meeting. Time will need to be allocated for the student to have a debriefing session with the clinical teacher on the conduct and outcome of the meeting and the student's own evaluation of their participation. The preparation of a written report by the

student is valuable in encouraging reflection on what happened – another item for the log book.

9. **Meetings with other students**. In some contexts, for example in a large hospital, there will be students from a range of professions. Opportunities could be explored for students from different disciplines to meet and perhaps work together. This is an excellent way to learn about team work; students having a positive experience of team work during their pre-registration course are likely to carry this into their professional practice.

10. **Plan graded steps to team involvement**. Having considered the level of difficulty of various elements of team work, grade the student involvement. For example, do not first of all send the student off to a case discussion with a consultant who never listens to what the 'paramedical team' has to say, or who fires questions at anyone around! Perhaps start with the student working alongside another member of the home team in group work with patients. Next, encourage the student to discuss a case with your most cooperative team member. Gradually work up to more demanding situations, e.g. case conferences, domiciliary work, school visits, collecting information from other team members, presentation at a case conference, etc.

11. **Gradually lead the student towards independence in team work**. At the student's first case conference, perhaps require him/her to contribute to the discussion of only one aspect of a patient's problem. Alternatively, get him/her to be responsible for speaking about one case, ensuring that this is not the first case to be discussed.

12. **Preparing reports and referrals**. Students cannot become competent at writing reports and letters in the classroom; such skills can only be developed fully in the work situation. Therefore, expect students to write letters of referral to other agencies as well as reports for the cases they are working with. Check the draft and countersign the final version. You will already have ensured that students have access to the same clinical information as the rest of the team. Also ensure that reports received from other team members are seen by the student. This needs to be monitored carefully, especially when a student is in the department only once a week.

13. **Explore ways information is passed on**. In addition to formal letters and reports, ensure that the student understands that communication can also take place through chats over coffee and 'phone calls. Remind the student about confidentiality.

14. **The team's time**. Encourage the student to respect the value of the time of other team members through time-keeping and prompt responses.

15. **Provide the student with opportunities for working alongside others:** Some pre-registration physiotherapy courses have the excellent practice

of requiring students to work in a hospital ward as part of the nurisng team. This must have a profound effect on the ability of physiotherapists to work effectively with nurses on qualification. Education students and speech and language therapy students have been given the opportunity of jointly assessing a child during their training (David and Smith, 1987). Leeds Polytechnic (1991, pers. commun.) brings together students from courses in education, health visiting, school nursing and speech and language therapy for a day to: 'involve the students in an interactive event which will present them with the opportunity to experience multidisciplinary education and provide them with a clearer understanding of each others roles and the potential for collaboration in the future'.

All professionals expect that new recruits will be able to work as team members, but perhaps we do not always do enough to give students from different fields the opportunity of working together. Many more opportunities for bringing together students from different fields in the working situation, need to be explored. Towards the end of a course it is important for a clinical teacher to evaluate whether he/she feels confident in a student's ability to work within the team, as well as to question if the student has been provided with all the requisite opportunities for learning to become an effective team member.

FOLLOW-UP ACTIVITIES

1. Examine the aims of observations on p. 92. Evaluate them in the context of your own field and, if appropriate, amend or extend them.
2. Take a list of the aims you have made and gradually identify the opportunities you could provide to enable students to achieve these aims. Examples are shown for two aims on p. 93–94. When you have done this, look at the list of observation opportunities on p. 107. Ensure that you have used all the appropriate opportunities. You will probably be able to add to the list. Your own list will be your learning resource. It is essential that the opportunities are used in relation to the aims/needs of the student.
3. Having considered the observation guidelines in this chapter, prepare some guidelines for students in your own clinical setting. Get some students to use and evaluate them.
4. Prepare a detailed teaching schedule for one of the procedures used in your work. Try this out with a student and ask them to evaluate the usefulness.
5. Examine the opportunities available in your own setting for the student to fit into the team. Ensure that these opportunities are explored for the students you work with.

6. Find out how many health care students are working in your locality.
7. Make a list of possible ways that students from your own field and students from other fields might work together. Try to follow up at least one of these ideas.

REFERENCES

Crago, M.B. and Pickering, M. (1987) *Supervision in Human Communication Disorders*, College Hill Press, Boston.

David, R. and Smith, B. (1987) Preparing for Collaborative Working, *British Journal of Special Education*, **14**, no. 1, 19–23.

Fish, D., Twinn, S. and Purr, B. (1990) *How to Enable Learning Through Professional Practice*. West London Institute of Higher Education in association with Brunel University.

National Health Service Training Authority (1987) Report of a Working Party on the *Development of Supervisors of Students in the Health Professions*.

Rassi, J. (1978) *Supervision in Audiology*, University Park Press, Baltimore.

6

Helping students develop insights and skills in management

Peter Richards

When a student becomes a member of a clinical group and shares in work experience, as an integral part of a planned programme of learning, he/she has to face considerable changes in the learning environment. If the student is to take full advantage of the experience, the clinical teacher will need to interpret the environment, so that opportunities can be exploited and threats and anxieties minimized.

The student is not simply expected to be a passive member of the clinical group, but needs to be an active member if the learning is to prove effective. The investment of the time and effort of the clinical teacher and colleagues needs to be made worthwhile. Learning will be accomplished best in this setting by 'doing' but only if the experiences are managed consciously and adequately structured.

Both students and teachers, at college and in the placement, will therefore need to be aware of the **management** aspects of this element of the curriculum. Each should be able to develop and practice appropriate skills which will lead towards increased effectiveness in the workplace. Each should benefit from an understanding of management processes. These should be able to be related to other situations, outside the immediate teaching and learning relationship. Evidence of mutual benefit will be sought to justify the placement dimension of the educational programme.

KEY AREAS IN THE CHAPTER

There are four key areas in which management insights and skills have to be developed:

1. Understanding the way formal organizations are structured; the way they are 'contrived' as systems to meet anticipated tasks and to respond

to expectations and conventions relevant to the particular sector of employment in which they are established.

2. Helping the teacher and learner to make the best use of the resources available; physical and human tools and energies, and to mobilize them for short- and long-term assignments. Planning for, allocating, monitoring and maintaining these resources and being accountable for their proper use.

3. Discovering and fulfilling a corporate role (or roles) within an organizational team. Identifying not only appropriate professional and technical contributions which can be made and recognized, but learning how individual personalities and behaviours can be accommodated into effective 'team working'.

4. Becoming more autonomous and independent as responsible individuals. Developing confidence and intuitive discretion as someone on whom others can depend. If someone is to be an effective manager of others, that person first needs to be able to manage him/herself and recognize the potential and the limitations which mark the thresholds of their own effective performance.

These key areas are all inter-related; they cannot be handled discretely in a strictly sequential manner. In this chapter we shall try, however, to set out some managerial guidelines for clinical teachers as if the areas were capable of being considered as separate topics.

USING MODELS TO HELP DESCRIBE COMPLEX REALITY

Describing the 'real world' in terms which are neatly packaged and labelled, identifying logical and identifiable causes and effects and pointing to clear patterns of relationships which are predictable are some of the challenges which face the clinical teacher. To make sense of organizational structures and processes in a way which will be of lasting value to the student, the teacher has to identify the everyday pragmatic world of professional practice. Models are useful shorthand concepts and tools to help to do this, but students and clinical teachers alike need to be aware of the difference between a 'model' or representation of reality and the pragmatic reality itself.

Students will already have learned a good deal about the theories of their discipline. They will have needed to learn many things in this idealized way. They will probably expect their work experience to coincide with the theories and models which they have been taught. It is very tempting, as a consequence, for the clinician to dismiss theories as 'academic' and thus to be dismissive of formal book knowledge, with the assertion that the student is 'in the real world now' and must start to learn again. To manage, and help the student to manage, this difficult transition clinical teachers must take steps to revise and re-emphasize the theoretical base for their own systems and procedures. Only then can there be a conscious relationship between the theoretical rationale for their practice and their pragmatism. This can be very demanding and requires patience and discipline.

LINKING THEORY AND PRACTICE

In helping the student to appreciate the significance of applying theory, not only will there be a tension between college-based learning and actual professional practice, but the clinician's own 'real-world' will also seem at variance from the formal organization in which they are said to work. Charts, tree diagrams, job descriptions (which are available to show to the student) can differ quite markedly from what might be the way things are organized in practice. The informal organizations can be just as real as the charts in the NHS 'management structure handbook'. Unless handled sensitively this apparent divergence between theory and practice can cause confusion and concern to the student. Follow-up activity 1 at the end of this chapter, suggests a way for the clinical teacher to carry out an exercise which could be very

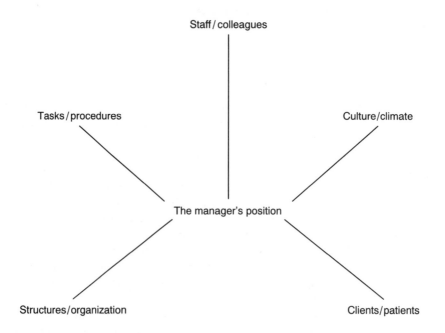

Figure 6.1 The manager's central position. After Walton (1984).

useful during the induction of a student into the way that organization is structured.

Students and clinicians need to be aware of the limitations of using Models as ways of presenting systems and procedures in a simplified and convenient manner. They can, however, be helpful aids in understanding the complexity of the real world. Managers will need to be familiar with modelling, not only as a way of describing and explaining how things work, but also as the basis for prediction and intervention, through planning, monitoring and control.

A simple diagramatic model for general reference, showing the way a manager's position can be seen in relation to activities and influences in their organization is set out in Fig. 6.1. Another model (Fig. 6.2) showing the

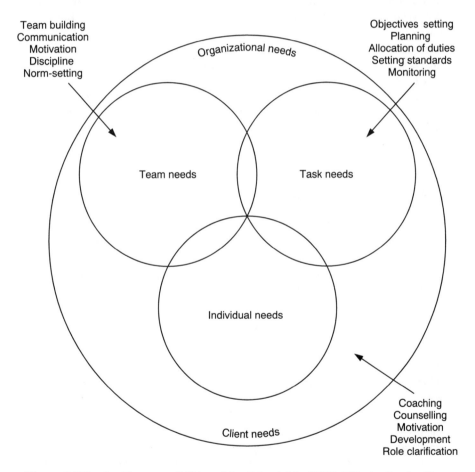

Figure 6.2 Leadership responsibilities. After John Adair (1983) *Effective Leadership*

inter-relationship between Task, Team and Individual has been suggested by Adair (1983). It is evident from this representation that significant tensions can arise from attempting to prioritize any one of the three concerns to the detriment of the others. Miller and Rice (1967), Paton *et al.* (1984) and Mintzberg (1983), provide further information on Organizations, Systems and Models.

Induction checklists

The student needs to be adequately briefed before joining in the work environment. Some of this briefing should take place in advance. This will be the joint responsibility of the placement tutor at the college and the host organization. Basic information about the location, access by public transport, correct postal addresses and telephone numbers of relevant staff, names and ranks of key individuals, size and nature of the unit, characteristics of the area and its population should be included. These ideas have been fully explored in Chapter 4.

An induction process is set up to assist the student to be more aware of the way things are done in the workplace. In the managerial context the induction can be used to illustrate how the manager needs to view things from a 'helicopter' perspective, to understand the way various people in the organization depend on each other and have to follow established procedures and channels of communication. A perspective which enables both an overview of operations and an ability to intervene quickly in incidents 'on the ground' when they occur.

Students will need to be introduced to the other members of staff as soon as possible upon arrival. Not only is this an appropriate courtesy, it is a mark of organizational efficiency for students and colleagues on the patch to know each other's names and designations and have an opportunity to establish a formal working relationship.

Role models of organizational behaviour

The quality of management will often only be evident in the detail of their day-to-day behaviour in the workplace. The clinical teacher will be modelling what is seen to be appropriate, ethical and cost-effective in the professional role. Consciously or unconsciously this will set the standard which the student is expected to follow and which reflects the acceptable relationship between the professional and the organization for mutual advantge. Attention to detail will begin to inform students on placement about organizations when they are at their most impressionable stage in professional development. The clinical teacher will become an influential role model and, although there will be other role models, the student will be quick to pick up cynicism, lack of commitment and integrity and inconsistency in behaviour.

Sometimes the clinical teacher will be looking out for actual examples of bad practice, these can then be used as powerful illustrations of what not to do.

Who to go to for help

Some of the most important checklists the student will require are the details of whom to go to in critical circumstances, such as times of personal stress or crisis, in handling complaints or grievance procedures, or in dealing with problems in working with a client. The teacher will be encouraging the student to work independently as much as possible, but there are times when it is important to ask for help and advice. There may also be times when it is right to refer a case or a problem to a specialist or to an office holder in higher authority. To the practitioner this may often seem to be an intuitive skill, but to the inexperienced newcomer these instances will need to be made explicit by setting out guidelines for practice.

A COMMUNICATION MAP

Most formal documentation about the structure and authority in an organization sets this out conventionally in the form of an hierarchy. Figure 6.3 illustrates a typical pattern of Management Hierarchy in a Health Authority, in the UK. In fact, in nearly all organizations, this is how authority and responsibility is described. Most formal communication also follows the horizontal and vertical lines of this hierarchical structure and authority. Indeed, potential problems may exist in ignoring the formal regularity of status and specialism in bureaucratic organizations: that is organizations whose dominant procedures follow the discipline of formal, published rules and conventions. A useful general text on Communications and Organizations can be found in Porter and Roberts (1977).

Sometimes, however, a formal picture of hierarchy may not be the most appropriate way of introducing the student to the organization of the workplace. So an alternative way of describing the communication pattern in an organization, as perceived by a particular member of that organization, is to set out a 'map' of those expected routes or connections which actually take place in the form of written or spoken communication; one example is shown in Fig. 6.4. In fact, the two forms of description of an organization are not so much alternative expressions of the same thing but important different perspectives from an individual or corporate viewpoint. They are both useful, therefore, in helping a student to understand the actual structures and processes

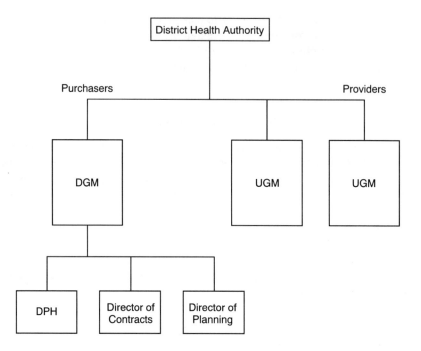

Figure 6.3 Management hierarchy in a health authority.

within the work environment. Various levels of sophistication can be developed to extend the detail of communication flows on such a map. Individuals may communicate, or receive different messages acting in different Roles in Fig. 6.4. The map could be elaborated greatly: the centre of the ring might be subdivided into role segments which an be projected into the outer circles. diagrammatic conventions such as arrows might indicate one- or two-way flows of information, predominance of the direction of flow or the initiation of the data; priorities can be indicated by the thickness of the connecting lines. If colour is used, different colours may refer to different kinds of communication; instruction, technical information, advice, referral, statistics and so on.

Influences on an organization

One advantage of a map is that it incorporates people and interests within the scope of the organization's influence, which might not be shown at all in formal charts. The links for example between the practitioner and the client, the general public, the media, other specialists in different organizations, the regulating bodies of government and of the profession, trade unions and so on. All of these are vitally important in the understanding of how a clinical practice operates and relates to its environment when seen from a manager's point of view. Learning about management requires both student and teacher to be much more aware of those wider influences upon an organization. This includes much that takes place outside the normal organizational boundaries of the clinic, hospital, school, etc.

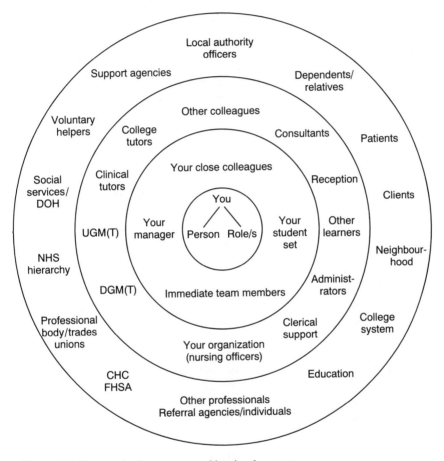

Figure 6.4 Communications map, working in placement.

THE MANAGEMENT OF RESOURCES

It will be an important contribution to a student's development if they can be exposed during their placement, to the harsh discipline of resource management within finite budgets. Learning about the financial aspects of care and the service is a vital part of the development of an effective practitioner. A general treatment of this issue in context is to be found in Fielding and Berman (1990). Other books on resource management and financial aspects are for example: Jones and Prowle (latest year); Perrin (1988) and Procter (1986). Great care needs to be exercised to refer to texts containing the latest arrangements and legislation for the National Health Service, in the UK and similar organizations elsewhere.

The earlier these financial concepts can be incorporated into the c·nsiderations which a professional will make in planning for a responsible regime for the client the better. It is unlikely that students will be given any direct responsibility either for establishing a budget or being made accountable for its operation. However it is useful if, during work experience, they are able to take some part in the planning, monitoring, cost-effectiveness and other evaluation processes which occur within the unit. Follow-up activity 2 in this chapter, may help the clinical teacher to prepare for a positive approach to managing within a tight economic environment. It may be necessary for a manager to test the apparent limits on resources by making a coherent and convincing case for additional resources (funds, time, personnel, equipment, etc.) It will sometimes be demonstrated that staff complaints and criticisms are actually unreasonable and that further resources are not justified. On the other hand, if a valid case can be made this will sometimes help in persuading the fund-holder to modify previous restrictions or provide the addditional resources needed.

Managing resources more effectively may sometimes mean neither increasing the output nor reducing the financial input required, but doing things differently with the same resources. Ways of allocating funds and of tying up budgets that may have been established earlier may need to be reconsidered from a cost-effective standpoint. For example, changes in demography, age-profile and employment patterns may influence whether times and venues for clinics may need to be changed for better attendance. Students could help clinicians by piloting sample questionnaires of preferred service provision. In doing this they will, at the same time, come to appreciate better the factors influencing the client's response in that local area.

Staffing

Students will need to learn the special language (jargon) of resource planning and control. Not only the use of relevant accounting terms used in management of the expenditure and the preparation of budgets, but terms and techniques in the planning and allocation and control of pesonnel. Students can be given the opportunity to see what takes place when task allocation occurs:

- Timetabling
- Establishment of duty rostas
- Holiday planning
- Covering arrangements for sickness
- Arranging for absences for other duties

It will be vital in management terms not only to see this as a necessary technical, numerate exercise, but to see how particular resources can be most effectively deployed in terms of specific, available expertise. It can also be used as a way of providing a varied staff experience in clinical situations.

Perhaps the clinical teacher, in planning the training programme for the student, might take advantage of there being a supernumerary person on the staff to enable the student (or indeed another colleague, as part of their management development) to attend a meeting of the Unit General Management Team, or even a meeting at Health Authority level. Even more, local meetings of the health and safety group, a quality circle or case conferences may provide insights into the process of formal meetings and the interests declared by other representatives of a multiprofessional or multi-agency network. The opportunity to attend, as observer, and be required to write up the proceedings critically, would be beneficial to any staff member seeking to discover more about management activities and pressures. Of course the cost-effectiveness itself of this additional use of resources needs careful consideration in the prevailing circumstances. Such activities and responsibility can often seem remote and irrelevant to the clinician, so an insight into what goes on, and what pressures managers are themselves under can be mutually helpful as well as instructive.

STAFF DEVELOPMENT

Follow-up activity 3 in this chapter, provides a further way for the clinical teacher to model an activity to be shared subsequently with a student. An aspect which this exercise draws out particularly is the importance of 'continuing professional development' for all qualified staff, based on an appraisal of existing skills and experience, and with a planned strategy for further enhancement. It may help the student to realize that there is no fundamental distinction between teacher and learner in development needs; it may demonstrate the continued importance of planned study at all stages of one's professional career. For further reference see Cox and Beck (1984) and Pedler *et al.* (1986).

A Strengths, Weaknesses, Opportunities and Threats (SWOT) analysis, as shown in Fig. 6.5, can be undertaken either for an individual member of staff of the team or for the unit as a whole. This may help to identify what

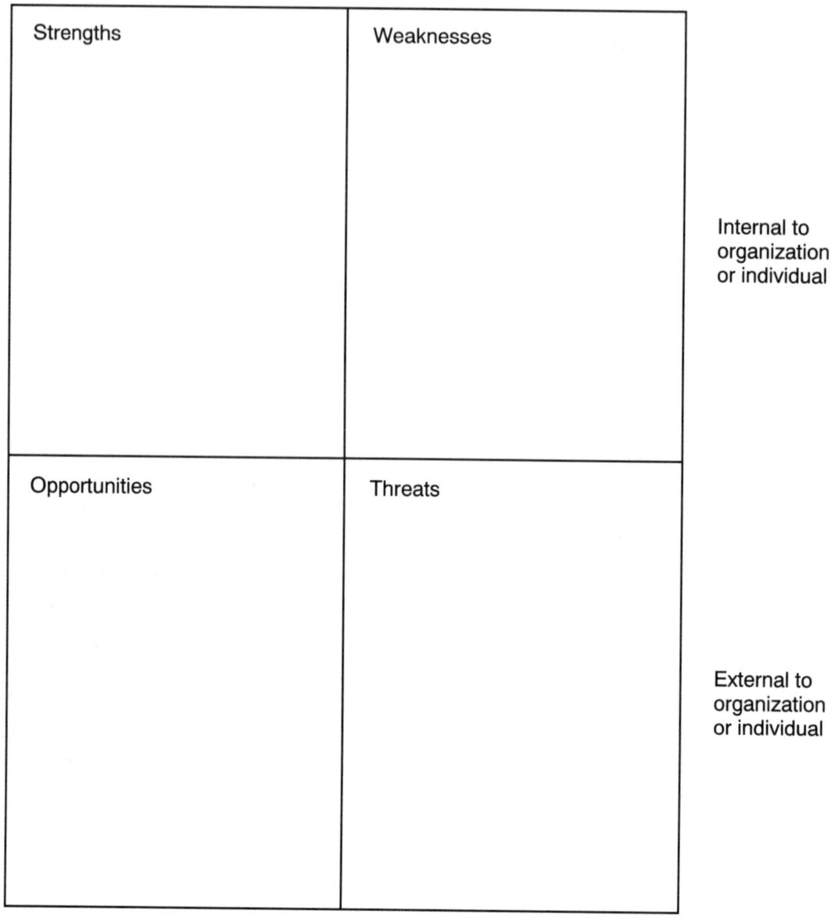

Strengths	Weaknesses	
		Internal to organization or individual
Opportunities	Threats	
		External to organization or individual

Figure 6.5 A SWOT analysis.

can be done to improve effective performance or to plan opportunities to take advantage of a changing situation. Weaknesses may be converted by managers into strengths and threats into opportunities through a skillful application of creative perception. Four key questions can be asked of apparently negative entries on the SWOT matrix:

1. Is this real or imagined?
2. Can this be inverted and treated as a positive advantage?
3. Can this be attended to by training?
4. Is this capable of being avoided or protected against?

An alternative exercise in self-assessment can be found in Walton (1984, p. 294).

TIME MANAGEMENT

Time in meetings, in waiting, in travelling, and so on can often appear to be wasted time. Effective time management is an expertise demanded of a competent clinician and is a key skill for managers. Time management courses are in great demand for management training, but there are some useful, informal things which can be done in the work place while a student is on placement. Such activities can help the newcomer as well as existing staff to use time more skilfully. In Fig. 6.6 a way of identifying time allocation is suggested.

A variant on this can be set out as a **job map**, showing the percentage of time or the priority ratings allocated to various tasks or roles; preferences or intentions to vary these allocations can be shown. This may be through delegation; it may involve a conscious self-discipline to try to correct an inbalance; it may even be useful as a starting point for personal appraisal within a structured Individual Performance Review (IPR) procedure with senior management. Useful further help can be found in Garratt (1985).

In a formal, structured, 'production' organization a great deal of time is carefully scheduled and allocated to specific tasks. If the organization were to 'work like clockwork' this would prove an efficient and effective use of available personnel. In 'service' organizations, rarely can all activities be anticipated or planned to that extent. Many situations arise which need to be managed spontaneously, for example:

1. urgent or emergency cases occur;
2. time allocated to appointments may need to be exceeded;
3. unforseen clinical or counselling matters arise which cannot be deferred;
4. transport may be late;
5. patients may not turn up when expected;
6. colleagues who were to have shared in a decision may be unavoidably involved elsewhere.

As a rule of thumb, only about 80% of the time can ever afford to be 'programmed' as routine, that is allocated in a strictly predictable manner and assumed to operate to that plan. About 20% of all time needs to be managed less predictably and made available to respond to unplannable issues which are bound to arise. These may in fact be the most important or urgent matters which require attention. For management scheduling this is especially the case and a simple measure of **efficiency** in planning the use of resources will be inadequate as a true measure of **effectiveness**. If space is not set aside for critical incidents to be managed then crises are likely to occur which interrupt the best organized programme.

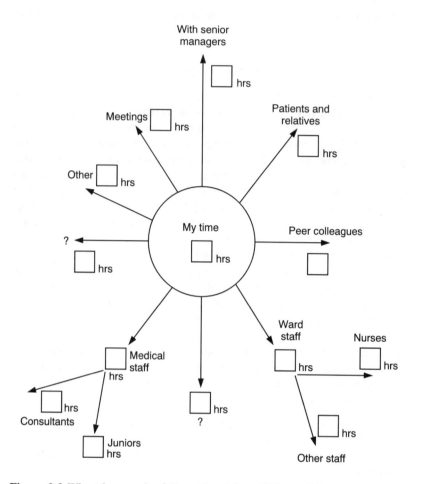

Figure 6.6 Who takes my time? Reproduced from Walton (1984), with permission.

Students need to be helped to appreciate the implications of formal quantitive measurement of programmable outcomes such as Korner statistics, but realize that sometimes the strict application of measurable data alone may not be the best assessment of achievement or effective use of resources.

Good management is characterized by an ability to handle uncertainty and ambiguity, and a willingness to appreciate that when things do not go exactly to plan this may in fact provide unforseen opportunities and advantages. In organizations, busy managers need to arrange things so that some space is also available within a busy routine for:

- Creative innovation
- Reading and research
- Reflection and critical assessment
- Forecasting and planning
- Social meetings
- Careful maintenance of human relationships

Such attitudes in dealing with contingencies and change may also require the manager more openly to admit the need for assistance and advice. It is a gracious manager who will, when appropriate, admit a lack of knowledge or of specific expertise and seek for the information or help from someone more knowledgeable. An admission of fallibility and a promise to 'find out' can be an endearing quality respected in management.

Meetings and more meetings

As management responsibility is devolved to the operational levels in an organization, staff planning meetings will become increasingly a feature of weekly and monthly programmes. These can be a distraction from clinical duties and can be considered a nuisance or a waste of time. It is important that clinical teachers and students learn to evaluate critically the way meetings are run and indeed the justification for these being held at all. It may help to develop a quality checklist as an aid to evaluate meetings:

1. timing;
2. location;
3. frequency;
4. agenda-building procedure;
5. content and level;
6. duration;
7. formality (e.g. in the way they are chaired);
8. reporting convention and detail.

Sometimes an outsider can be used to provide objective and yet sensitive feedback to a group's overall performance and help to use time more effectively. Colleagues from different departments or sections can often help each other reciprocally, without knowing the detailed content of the business.

Diaries and log books

The crucial discipline of keeping and using a diary or log book is something which both student and teacher ought to reinforce; their use was discussed in earlier chapters. It is probable that the student will have been encouraged to maintain a record of learning experiences in which activity and identified learning need will have been set down regularly. This kind of record will be very helpful also during a placement. It could include:

1. specific targets and objectives;
2. a detailed record of what the student has been asked to do;
3. how the duties were performed;
4. what plans or opportunities for further experience were identified during practice;
5. an assessment of the appropriateness of the training plan;
6. some clear statements of achieved competence.

Keeping records is a necessary professional discipline. Patient case records, ward records and clinical notes are all part of accepted care planning. It is just as important to maintain records of personal learning and development.

Managers are notoriously poor at maintaining a trail or back-up record of past events (e.g. complaints) for subsequent analysis; they are often too eager, once a case has been dealt with, to press on to the next; this action-orientation fails to exploit the lessons learnt from experience as fully as possible. The importance of reflection as part of the total learning experience has already been stressed in many aspects of the student's learning experience.

The requirement for the student to maintain a diary or a log book is sometimes treated only as an assessment requirement. The record should prove invaluable in constructing a curriculum vitae (CV). It may be the source of evidence to demonstrate the attainment of specific competencies within training and may form part of a portfolio of demonstrated experience and achievement. A discipline such as this may in fact be helpful to initiate what is hoped might be a regular, longer-term commitment in professional practice after qualification.

The clinical teacher can use the student's diary as:

- A basis for planning
- For counselling and tutorial help
- For further vocational training
- For career advice
- To identify the potential strengths and weaknesses in a student's proven competence

It also makes the move towards regular Individual Performance Review (as part of continuing professional development) a lot less threatening than it is sometimes seen at present.

LEARNING ABOUT ROLES IN ORGANIZATIONS

There is a strong element of artificiality in organizations. As we saw at the start of this chapter, organizations are systems, contrived (designed) to fulfil particular objectives or to meet specific needs. The larger the organization and the more complex, the greater the tendency towards 'mechanistic' or highly structured forms which are far from 'natural' in the way people are used to achieve tasks. Bureaucratic organizations tend to use individuals to fill role slots; people are appointed to posts or offices in which much of their natural personality is submerged by the formalized behaviour and activity consistent with that role. It is likely therefore that in formal organizations individuals will see their contributions primarily in terms of their technical activity; their skills and abilities will be measured against task targets or professional work criteria. It is important for managers to enable individuals, within a structure such as the NHS to be able to contribute from their personal characteristics their identified strengths and weaknesses and natural abilities as well.

Role behaviour

There is always a kind of tension between role behavour and the authentic autonomous behaviour natural to an individual. This tension is more tolerable at the operational level in an organization where individuals can gain primary satisfaction from the task. At managerial levels individuals look additionally for personal satisfaction and an identity with the service as a fulfillment of themselves. They are less likely, or able, to end the day and switch off from work to a different 'personal' life. Managers therefore need to consider carefully the demands and opportunities presented by the roles demanded of a particular position holder and seek to negotiate, or accommodate, to a form of the role which best equates with the individual's talents and potential for the future.

When helping a student to take up a new professional career the clinical teacher may be very influential in establishing a 'role identity' for the clinician. What the student first learns to label as expected attitudes and behaviours can have lasting consequences for the commitment and fulfillment of that individual in the service. Students may have to learn the difficult lesson that their 'idol', who has formed their role model, cannot always be copied, if they are to be authentic and effective as themselves.

Management roles

The clinician may have to think carefully about his/her own changing role as a teacher and manager. Mintzberg (1973) identified 10 key roles for a typical manager:

- Figurehead
- Leader
- Liaison
- Monitor
- Disseminator
- Spokesperson
- Entrepreneur
- Resource allocator
- Disturbance handler
- Negotiator

Rarely does a manager relate to one role alone. A role-set is made up of distinctive 'character parts' which you expect to act in different situations. It may form quite a complex set of behaviours a manager may need to exhibit in an organization. Some roles will be related to an internal situation within the work setting; others will affect the way one presents oneself, as a representative, to the outside world. Walton (1984) shows an example, related to the Health Service, of a complex role set (Fig. 6.7). Further study could be pursued in Stewart (1989) and Lawton and Rose (1991).

Role-holders may rank the relative importance and the relative amount of time spent in each role quite differently. It would be a useful exercise (see Jauch *et al.*, 1983) for students to carry out interviews with various managers (ideally both inside and outside the Health Service). They will need to discover the relative *time* that each person believes they spend fulfilling each of these roles and the relative *priority* or importance of the role to their organizational effectiveness. They will inevitably come across differences and conflicting perceptions in the way different managers in different levels of the hierarchy, and carrying out different functions, prioritize their roles. Students can then compare the results of their interviews, either on placement or after return to college, and try to understand the rationale behind such differences. They may be able to discover a pattern which will help them to appreciate why managers respond in a particular way to identifiable situations.

Tests of the extent to which a person is bound into the limitations of any role can be made by asking them searching questions about:

- What one has to do (demands)
- What one is prevented from doing (constraints)
- What one can choose to do (choices/options)

There is nearly always an area of negotiated discretion around the core of the role as it is defined by the system.

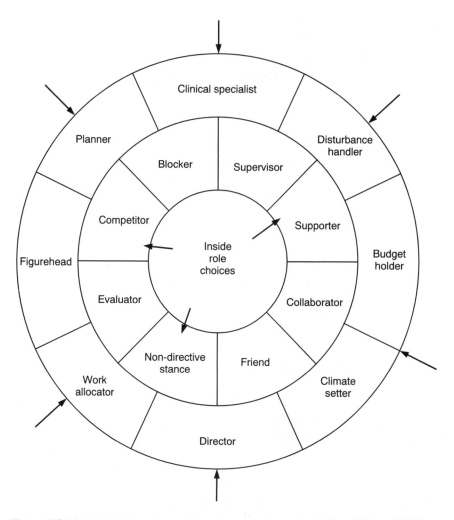

Figure 6.7 Inside choices and external requirements. Reproduced form Walton (1984), with permission.

Plant (1987) looks at the way the role you are allocated, or carve out for yourself in the organization, has a considerable impact on your ability to influence your surroundings. Some people only operate in a small central area of their role, which can be called a 'zone of comfort' (Fig. 6.8). Managers may need to extend the scope of their role and so step outside this zone to

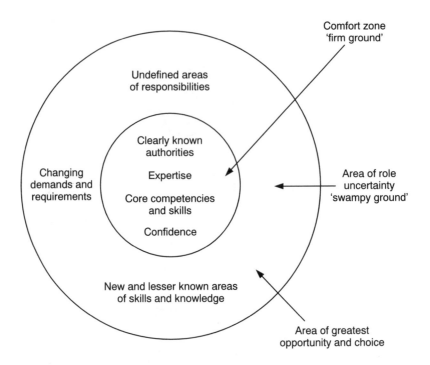

Figure 6.8 Aspects of role. Reproduced from Plant (1987), with permission.

the less safe but more rewarding area beyond. We shall see below that key skills in management will include assertiveness and the willingness to take risks.

The use of role play

Role-play techniques may be helpful in developing managerial skills as well as to make one more familiar with other people's expectation of role. The clinical teacher can help to set up appropriate situations and coach the student to act out the role of a clinician in a particular situation. This type of role-play exercise could also usefully be introduced in the college setting, and was referred to in Chapter 2. Role playing can also be undertaken by colleagues (or other students) to represent typical client behaviour. This should be in a safe context and help the student to rehearse an anticipated situation, in order to develop techniques and confidence. Care should be taken not to over-exaggerate or stereotype roles unduly and thus reduce the sense of reality. On the other hand, some management development specialists argue the benefits of drama and fantasy in role play to gain depths of understanding which are hidden by more self-conscious forms of analysis. Goffman (1956) for example, shows how people can present 'masks' to the world and can not only hide their true selves from others but also from themselves. These concepts are familiar to those health care professionals who frequently use counselling in their treatment of patients.

The understanding of the psychological effects and consequences of changes of role, in times of organizational change or reorganization, are especially valuable to students during placements. They may be going themselves through a profound change of role and responsibility and will be more conscious of the effects on tutors and clinical teachers. The NHS also is going through an extended time of organizational change; insights into the nature of changes, for the Service as well as for individuals will contribute to all those coping with the trauma of change and help them to manage more positively. As well as Plant (1987) other sources are Mayon-White (1986), Handy (1989) and Carnall (1990).

Roles in teamwork

Much has been written about the importance of teams and teamwork in organizations. The devolution of responsibility in the NHS has made the development of effective management teams possible and now even more important. Management is both a responsibility of individuals holding key posts and of corporate groups sharing in:

- Controlling
- Coordinating
- Planning
- Motivating
- Organizing
- Directing
- Rewarding
- Reviewing
- Setting standards

The student, during work experience, joins an existing team and will have an influence on the way that team works. Teams are transient and need to be capable of taking on and losing members, quickly re-establishing their effective performance. There are well-researched phases of team development where typical behaviour and relationships between members can be observed. Tuckman (1965) sets out the stages: forming; storming; norming; performing and adjourning as identifiable phases through which groups, acting as teams, are likely to go. At each phase they are likely to face anticipated difficulties, and moving from one phase to the next may pose particular crises.

The student will probably want to join the team and be recognized and valued as an active participant. Being part of a team may also provide an opportunity to learn by observing the behaviour of a real working group from the inside and reflect on what takes place. Any interventions and insights will need to be facilitated by a knowledgeable and sensitive teacher aware of group processes.

Teams depend on members providing mutual support; they are more flexible in their performance of specific tasks than other organizational forms and there is less demarcation by discrete specialisms. However, specialist contributions are called for and team members need to identify and be accepted for the specialisms they offer. The factor of size may need to be considered, sometimes teams may grow too large for identity or for the effective allocation of roles. Teams may need to subdivide for all or part of their work. Such differentiation can call on extra management effort and skill for integration. Some specialisms will coincide with professional status and training, but team members will not always act in their formal status in relationships with one another. Particular specialist contributions may also be offered on the basis of skills and attributes not formally recognized or demanded in the job specification, e.g. artistic talents, gifts of salesmanship, public speaking, critical assessment, empathy, etc. Belbin (1981) identifies eight key team roles, based on a personality profile or inventory as:

- Company worker (CW)
- Chairman (CH)
- Shaper (SH)
- Resource investigator (RI)
- Monitor evaluator (ME)
- Team worker (TW)
- Completer finisher (CF)
- Plant (PL)

A useful exercise for individuals to test which roles are most, and least, suitable will be found in the same publication. Clinical teachers might find the exercise valuable for themselves as well as for students.

Individuals can make powerful personal contributions as: ideas generators, time-keepers, devil's advocates, jokers and tension diffusers. A sacrificial role can sometimes be an ultimate contribution; a scapegoat to carry the guilt can enable a team to go on surviving even in spite of a past catastrophe.

The student's attributes of recent academic knowledge and theoretical insights can be considered as a threat or be explicitly acknowledged by using those contributions in committees or team development sessions. This may reinforce the value of earlier college-based learning and provide credibility and a sense of real belonging in practice.

Team leadership

Leadership in teams is not always undertaken as a role by the designated team manager or chairperson. Leadership will often emerge in the group, to be taken up by the person best suited in terms of particular knowledge, skill or experience in a specific situation. Leadership can also be deliberately rotated in order to help develop staff in leadership skills, where these may not be able to be practised or tested in other circumstances. The student may be given responsibility for leadership in certain chosen situations, provided there is backing and encouragement from other members of the team, prepared to make this possible. For example a student could be given responsibility for planning the management of a case with other professionals as part of the team.

The crucial importance of 'leadership' in the NHS is explored in Stewart (1989). She shows that it is a characteristic, supplementary to management, required at all levels of responsibility.

LEARNING ABOUT STYLES IN MANAGEMENT

There is no one way to be an effective manager. However we can all benefit by thinking about how we function and identify the options and alternative ways of managing.

Walton, 1984 (p.5)

Different styles of management and of leadership are evident in different organizations. The clinical teacher will need to help the student to learn about management and managing without being distracted by the stereotyping effect one particular style can have on the definition of the function of management as a whole.

Different styles are relevant to differing circumstances and will be instrumental in achieving particular outcomes through different approaches and strategies. Tannenbaum and Schmidt (1958) have suggested a continuum of managerial styles which provide us with a language to describe the relationship between the manager and the managed in terms of 'problem' ownership (Fig. 6.9). Even though the manager carries responsibility and is accountable for outcomes within his or her domain, the involvement of others in decisions and in implementing activity is at their discretion and a consequence of the style felt to be most appropriate.

In the NHS the extreme styles at either end of this continuum can be labelled 'autocratic' or '*laissez faire*'. Sometimes these are not helpful terms since

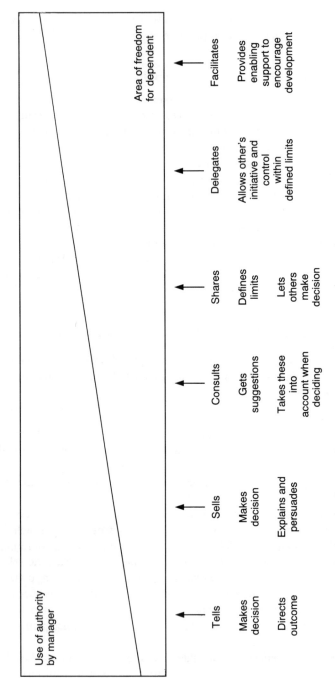

Figure 6.9 Continuum of leadership behaviour. Adapted from Tannenbaum and Schmidt (1958).

they tend to suggest an overall demeanour unrelated to the particular purpose for which the style or attitude is adopted. It might be more helpful to view the left-hand end of the continuum (Fig. 6.9), as that adopted principally by the expert or the specialist, in circumstances where they are assumed to know or have power or authority to decide, while the recipients of the 'directions' or 'orders'are ignorant or weak. It is a powerful hierarchical relationship in management based on rights to manage and rights to decide.

At the other end of the continuum is the style adopted principally by counsellors. The intention of this style is to help the client undertake responsibility for their own problems; this relationship will be familiar to many professionals working in health care. The characteristic management style is directed towards facilitating the client's development or releasing them from inhibitions caused by undue dependence. It is no less positive a style in that, correctly used, it can force a disadvantaged or weak individual to take initiatives which otherwise would tend to be avoided.

At other points of the continuum, various strategies of actual or token participation in decision-making are adopted. 'Selling' the decision retains ownership and power in the hands of the manager but allows the other person to feel their interests have been recognized. The centre ground is taken up with various forms of active participation. Throughout, the manager determines the basis of the relationship but response is needed from the subordinate before that style can be made effective. If the style is not carried off well, or if it is inappropriate in the situation, it is fairly easy to block the intended outcomes; this makes the strategy ineffective. Generally those being managed in organizations seek some consistency and rationality in the way different styles are employed; too wide a range of styles from one individual manager is difficult to sustain authentically. It also takes quite a little preparation and the development of trust to wean 'subordinates' away from a traditional inclination towards dependency and subservience.

Students should be given an opportunity to explore a range of situations, in which different styles are consciously adopted. This will increase their appreciation of the potential richness of the managerial approach. On the other hand they can be badly served by dogmatic or inflexible leadership behaviour.

DOMINANT ORGANIZATIONAL CULTURES

Adoption of roles and styles and the establishment of a characteristic structure for an organization is the product of the dominant culture or set of values and beliefs in that institution or sector. This culture will have developed and become entrenched over time. What is right, best or appropriate, particularly affecting corporate outcomes, will often be assumed without challenge.

Implicit priorities and biases can be identified by outsiders but are sometimes not evident to those within the system.

Handy (1978) has written about characteristically identifiable organizational cultures which exist in the Western World. It is useful to explore the definitions and illustrations of his four principle types of culture so as to be more aware of the characteristics and implications of one's own values and assumptions. Harrison (1972) offers some challenging opportunities to rethink one's basic ideologies about what is necessary and possible within organizational relationships. These writers identify stereotypes and major cultural orientations towards Power, Role, Task or Person.

A problem can arise if the values or background culture of an individual is widely at variance with the organization where he or she works. At the least, it will cause concern and a period of reorientation while settling in; at the worst, values and ideologies (especially at the ethical or political extremes), may prove irreconcilable. Hurt, anger or open conflict can result. The choices to get out of an unacceptable environment, to remain and suffer or to subvert and attempt to change the existing order, will each have significant consequences for both individual and organization. The clinical teacher needs to realize that this tension between the student's and organization's values and attitudes will be at its most critical point during an early period of work placement.

Particular attention may need to be paid to those from other ethnic or national backgrounds who may find indigenous customs and attitudes strange and unfamiliar. Gender stereotyping also needs to be watched in certain professional groups where one sex predominates; just as the special needs of women entering management positions should also be taken into account while they accommodate to what can be predominantly a male culture. Students may need these innate conflicts to be drawn to their attention and be helped to study strategies to ensure equal opportunities.

Follow-up activity 4 provides a framework for your own views and the views of other people in the organization to be explored more objectively and analytically. The questionnaire developed by Harrison (in Handy's *Understanding Organizations* (1978, Chapter 7)), could be used.

HELPING THE STUDENT TO GREATER INDEPENDENCE

The clinical teacher will be expected to help the student not only to learn about management but to help them actually manage. The concept of 'managing' for those who do not hold a formal title or carry the status of manager is important to grasp.

Managing is not only fulfilling a position in organizations related to power, authority and the responsibility, or for taking charge of people and facilities, it occurs as a process at all levels. Managing is not, in any case, restricted to formal organizations. People need to manage in all kinds of different circumstances and therefore there is some sense in which managing is a universal concept (Pedler and Boydell, 1985). Managing is integral to the work of all health care professionals; it is essential that students learn to recognize its aspects as part of their clinical responsibility.

There are some useful distinctions to be made between those who manage and those who are managed in organizations. There are characteristics of the management process which can generally be recognized even if opportunities to manage are few and far between. For those who are called to manage for a greater proportion of their time the characteristics which distinguish what they are expected to do are even more apparent. Here are a suggested set of characteristics which distinguish those who manage:

- Achieving tasks via others
- Organizing and preparing for the future
- Administering rules and procedures
- Coping with uncertainty (and relishing it!)
- Exercising discretion and judgement
- Maintaining organizational relationships.

It may be that the implications of these characteristics should be considered carefully by any clinicians considering undertaking managerial responsibilities themselves.

Managing on behalf of others

There is, however, a distinction which needs to be drawn between those who have to manage themselves in private settings, where the idea of being autonomous and independent predominates, from those in organizations where management is not so much about independence but about interdependence on others in a formal setting.

Managers in organizations have to act as agents for the corporate whole. They receive their status and their authority but, as a result, carry equivalent accountability and are responsible or answerable for their actions. This is so at all levels; their managing is therefore on behalf of some higher authority who ultimately directs and judges their performance. Sometimes this activity is described as administration; the differentiation is very rarely clear-cut but recognition of emphasis may be helpful (Stewart, 1989).

Managing learning

During their time in college, students should have been encouraged to undertake personal responsibilities for their studies; to manage their own learning. Their dependence on tutors and lecturers will need to have been reduced from the outset of a pre-qualification course and care will have been necessary even in quite small matters, to build up attitudes and environments in which students can be taught how to learn independently. The importance of independent, self-motivated learning in the developing professional has already been discussed earlier in this volume.

In a workplace setting this enabling relationship between learner and teacher can be reinforced. From the start of the placement the role of the clinical teacher needs to be worked through quite explicitly. A parent–child relationship is inappropriate. The student can be inhibited from having to work out ways of coping for themselves by teachers showing undue parental concerns, often with the very best of intentions. This does not imply that the students should be simply left to their own devices, but care is needed in structuring situations so as to provide a safe, supportive environment where the student has as much freedom as the situation allows. The teacher also has to be prepared to take the potential consequences of a sudden switch in behaviour, from dependence to counter-dependence, when at a critical phase a student turns from being reliant on the clinical teacher to overtly rejecting and devaluing that support. This can be personally difficult for the teacher to accept and the hurt of rejection can be experienced at the time. These aspects of the clinical teacher's role and the related problems were discussed in Chapter 3.

Managing and coping

Coping can sometimes be a useful synonym for managing; students will need to learn that in management much of the time those people are expected to achieve given objectives and targets with just that support which is available at the time. Managing means:

coping with inadequate *resources, information, time, preparation,*
coping with an inadequate *system/organization, boss*; *colleagues/team*; and
coping with one's inadequate *self.*

But accepting this is where you have to start.

Not to make a spectacular success of this is 'surprisingly' commonplace! In fact, when one thinks about it, it is not at all surprising that managers do not succeed all the time. Students and teachers need to be aware of realistic expectations in themselves and organizations. Clinicians will often judge management performance from their own criteria for achievement; this can be unfair and unhelpful.

Coping can sometimes mean just getting through the day; and it can be a way of thinking on one's feet. There has, nevertheless, to be a sensitive balance between dealing with the immediate and pressing contingencies and taking a detached, broader and longer-term view; to plan for the future and appreciate the patterns which are constant against those which are changing; this is also to cope.

Coping demands a positive and pro-active attitude to situations which might otherwise seem daunting. Achieving perfect solutions is rarely possible for managers, who may have set their sights instead on reaching adequate outcomes or surviving within acceptable limits. The concept of sufficiency or satisfying rather than maximizing is one for managers to appreciate (Cyert and March, 1963).

Management is not just about coping with daily uncertainty, risk, and being opportunistic and entrepreneurial. It is, above all, a political activity where what is right at one time will depend on key interested parties, all of whom one cannot please all the time. What is right for one can often be detrimental to another and viewed by that other interest as wrong.

Students may have a difficult psychological jump to make accepting that many of the things which go on in a clinical setting are measured less unambiguously and critically, in terms of right outcomes, than might have been imagined from an academic viewpoint. The teacher will need to encourage and counsel the student to appreciate this kind of managerial pragmatism without rejecting the standards established because of professional criteria. The parallel between this and the models of organization theory have already been noted earlier in this chapter.

HELPING TO BUILD MANAGEMENT SKILLS

Skills of managing are not exclusive to management; the same skills are often required in the effective performance of other duties. It is useful however to cluster certain skills, which can be practised and developed, focused on particular management activities. Then to recognize the transferable benefits of these skills in other areas of working life. Some skills identified already with existing professionalism in the Health Service may need to be modified and redirected as they are applied to management tasks. Skills associated with counselling, for example, are generic skills, as are those of communication and problem solving, but they take on a special relevance in management situations. The development of generic skills has been referred to in earlier chapters.

Lewis and Kelly (1986) have produced a very useful collection of activities designed to raise awareness and proficiency in applying the skills to a managerial situation (Box 6.1). Self-study workbooks (like Lewis and Kelly's), are recommended to the clinical teachers for use within the workplace.

Box 6.1 Twenty activities for developing managerial effectiveness. Reproduced from Lewis and Kelly (1986)

Communication skills
  Making meetings work
  Writing results
  Instructing subordinates
  Dealing with subordinates' problems
  Constructive questioning
Leadership skills
  Developing effective groups
  Delegating
  Being assertive
  Motivating subordinates
  Handling problem subordinates
  Managing change
  Handling conflict
Decision-making and problem-solving skills
  Deciding how to decide
  Identifying and analysing problems
  Generating solutions
  Getting decisions implemented
  Managing time.

Activities are planned to be undertaken within a work environment with the minimum of special equipment and overhead cost in time. Other examples of self development literature are Woodcock and Francis (1982), Stubbs (1986) and Pedler *et al.* (1986).

Skills can be developed by identifying the basic elements from which competences are made, such as:

- Assertiveness
- Listening
- Ability with numbers
- Memory
- Organizing things into categories
- Seeing relationships and patterns

These micro-skills can be practised, rather like playing scales on a musical instrument, as a preliminary to building up a broader set of proficiencies which can be put together into macro-skills.

Many management skills are related to performing effectively in inter-personal situations and require considerable insights into the way people behave and can be motivated. There may be a fine dividing line between persuading people to do something in the common interest and manipulating people against their will. Many of the skills can also in fact be thought of as political skills and sensitivities; these enable the manager to be perceptive and influential in integrating a variety of interests, often at variance with one another. A manager needs to be able to live with the consequences of using power and be prepared to enjoy as well as play the politics of a wider system. Politics may be considered to constitute one among a number of systems of influence of authority.

> Ideologies, and expertise may be described as legitimate in some sense. The system of politics by contrast may be described as reflecting power which is technically illegitimate as it is neither formally authorised, widely accepted or officially certified. . . .
>
> Mintzberg, 1983

Figure 6.10 maps a set of skills for managers as a series of overlapping circles; each could be thought to contain a cluster of related skills which might be given a generic label. When one looks closer one can see that skills in each circle are actually made up in combinations, between circles to the left and right. Thus real 'managing' skills are not discrete and clearly defined, they are subtle blends of perception and adroitness of technical ability, personal sensitivity and political astuteness.

The clinical teacher and the student will need to work together to develop skills by finding opportunities for practice in the context of work. If direct opportunities in the workplace cannot be made available to practice specific skills, the student should at least be encouraged to make observations about the make-up of management skills which they can identify around them. This will heighten their awareness not only of what these skills are, but how they are constructed and can be developed. Working situations should be as typical as possible in order to represent an experience consistent with that likely when the student becomes qualified.

As we set out at the start of this chapter, the clinical teacher needs to establish identifiable work assignments, typical enough to be modelled as good examples and yet natural enough to be part of the real world of clinical practice. If this can be achieved, students will benefit from the experience both of the understanding and the practice of management. The disciplined development of transferable managing skills will be of considerable benefit to both teacher and learner, as well as to the development and maintenance of effective and efficient health care provision for the whole organization.

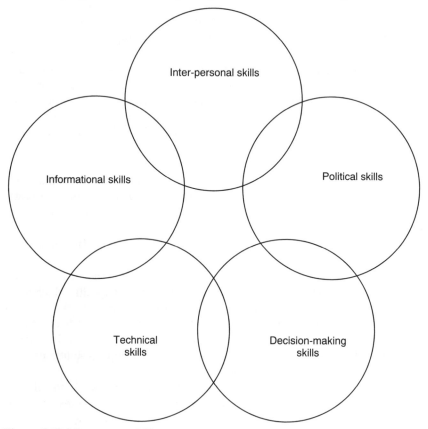

Figure 6.10 Management skills.

FOLLOW-UP ACTIVITIES

The following activities, although designed to be undertaken by the clinical teacher, are intended to enhance the practising of management skills, which will then be more usefully modelled in working with students.

1. Draw up a detailed organizational chart showing responsibilities and communication flows. Compare what should happen according to formal statements of job description and grading and what actually happens in a typical situation. Fit your clinic or practice into the wider context of the Health District and note the interdependencies in the service you provide.
2. Prepare a case, to be presented both orally and as a written report, for some additional funding for a specific item of expenditure which you consider justified. Use the conventions required in your Authority and see how these help or hinder your advocacy.

3. Carry out an audit of the skills and experience available of human resources upon which you can draw to help you accomplish your management tasks. Suggest training and development strategies to help you overcome the shortfall in existing resources which you decide are necessary for the enhancement of the service for which you are responsible.
4. Make a critical comparison of the values, attitudes norms and expectations evident in your organization's dominant culture with your own beliefs and behaviour preferences. What are you going to do about it? Can you think of ways that this might influence your career planning?

REFERENCES

Adair, J. (1983) *Effective Leadership – a self-development manual*, Gower Publishing, Aldershot, UK.

Belbin, R. (1981) *Management Teams – why they succeed or fail*, William Heinemann, London.

Carnall, C.A. (1990) *Managing Change in Organizations*, Prentice-Hall, Hemel Hempstead, UK.

Cox, C. and Beck, J. (eds) (1984) *Management Development – Advances in Practice and Theory*, John Wiley, Chichester.

Cyert, R.M. and March, J.G. (1963) *A Behavioral Theory of the Firm*, Prentice-Hall, Englewood Cliffs, New Jersey.

Fielding, P. and Berman, P.C. (eds) (1990) *Surviving in General Management – a resource for Health Professionals*, Macmillan Education, Basingstoke, UK.

Garratt, S. (1985) *Manage Your Time*, Fontana Paperbacks, London.

Goffman, E. (1956) *The Presentation of Self in Everyday Life*, Doubleday, London.

Handy, C.B. (1978) *Understanding Organizations*, Penguin Books, Harmondsworth, UK.

Handy, C.B. (1989) *The Age of Unreason*, Hutchinson, London.

Harrison (1972) How to Describe your Organization, *Harvard Business Review*, Sept–Oct.

Jauch, L.R., Coltrin, S.A., Bedeian, A.G. and Gluek, W.F. (1983) *The Managerial Experience – Cases, Exercises and Readings*, The Dryden Press, Chicago.

Jones, T. and Prowle, M. (latest year), *Health Service Finance an Introduction*, Certified Accountants Educational Trust.

Lawton, A. and Rose, A. (1991) *Organisation and Management in the Public Sector*, Pitman, London.

Lewis, M. and Kelly, G. (1986) *20 Activities for Developing Managerial Effectiveness*, Gower Publishing, Aldershot, UK.

Mayon-White, B. (ed.) (1986) *Planning and Managing Change*, Harper and Row, London (with Open University).

Miller, E.J. and Rice, A.K. (1967) *Systems of Organization*, Tavistock Publications, London.

Mintzberg, H. (1973) *The Nature of Managerial Work*, Harper and Row, New York.

Mintzberg, H. (1983) *Structure in Fives – designing effective organization*, Prentice-Hall, Englewood Cliffs, New Jersey.

Paton, R., Brown, S., Spear, R. *et al.* (eds) (1984) *Organizations – Cases, Issues, Concepts*, The Open University, Milton Keynes.

Pedler, M. and Boydell, T. (1985) *Managing Yourself*, Fontana, London.

Pedler, M., Burgoyne, J. and Boydell, T. (1986) *A Manager's Guide to Self Development*, 2nd edn, McGraw-Hill, Maidenhead, UK.

Perrin, J. (1988) *Resource Management in the N.H.S.*, Van Nostrand Reinhold with Health Service Management Centre, Birmingham.

Plant, R. (1987) *Managing Change and Making it Stick*, Fontana, London.

Porter, L.W. and Roberts, K.H. (eds) (1977) *Communication in Organizations*, Penguin Books, Harmondsworth, UK.

Procter, R. (1986) *Finance for the Perplexed Executive*, Fontana, London.

Stewart, R. (1989) *Leading in the NHS – a Practical Guide*, Macmillan Press, Basingstoke, UK.

Stubbs, R. (1986) *Assertiveness at Work*, Pan Books, London.

Tuckman, B.W. (1965) Developmental Sequences in Small Groups. *Psychological Bulletin*, **63**, 384–99.

Tannenbaum, R. and Schmidt, W. (1958) How to Choose a Leadership Pattern, in *Harvard Business Review*, March–April.

Walton, M. (1984) *Management and Managing – a Dynamic Approach*, Harper and Row, London.

Woodcock, M. and Francis, D. (1982) *The Unblocked Manager – a pracical guide to self development*, Gower Publishing, Aldershot, UK.

7

Feedback

INTRODUCTION

In this chapter the importance of feedback is stressed as a central tool for teaching and learning in the workplace. The why, how, when and where of feedback is thoroughly explored. As visits to students, by tutors from the course, are a major forum for feedback, the nature, content and difficulties of these visits will also be considered.

THE IMPORTANCE OF FEEDBACK TO PROMOTE LEARNING

One of the most effective ways of helping health care students to progress towards professional competence, is through the provision of clear and regular feedback (Warrender, 1990). There are a number of ways in which this takes place. In college, feedback is provided through such means as the comments made by tutors on written work, as well as on the student's ability to carry out procedures in practical situations, such as in workshops and clinical simulation exercises. However, the clinical teacher is in a unique position in being able to provide precise feedback to individual students on all aspects of professional development. It is only in the real work context that the teacher can see how the knowledge and skills worked up in college, are actually used.

Neville and French (1991) gathered views from physiotherapy students and clinical tutors on what constitutes 'good' or 'poor' clinical experience. All the students rated highly the provision of frequent, constructive feedback from their clinical tutors as a feature of 'good clinical experience'. There is no reason to think that physiotherapy students are unique in their views. Discussions with students from several fields indicates that they all see feedback as very important, but usually feel that they do not have enough.

Earlier we referred to the work of Argyris and Schon (1974) and noted their claim that each individual needs to have the opportunity to develop their own 'theories-of-action'. For these to be appropriate to the sphere of professional practice, students must be provided with a clear account of how they are doing. Although the key person in the feedback process is the clinician with whom the student is working, there are also some other ways in which feedback on clinical progress can be made available. These include:

- Feedback from self
- Feedback from peers
- Feedback from college tutors

WHAT IS FEEDBACK?

Ende (1983) provides a most useful definition in his paper on clinical feedback in clinical medical education. He defines it as 'information that a system uses to make adjustments in reaching a goal' and stresses that

the importance of feedback in the acquisition of skills follows from the nature of the clinical method. As a compendium of cognitive, psychomotor and affectual behaviours, clinical skills is easier demonstrated than described. And, like ballet, it is best learned in front of a mirror. Feedback occurs when a student is offered insight into what he/she actually did as well as the consequences for his/her actions.

Ende's definition immediately identifies several major points which we need to consider further.

1. In talking about adjustments in reaching a goal, he implies that feedback is not the same as evaluation or assessment, the endpoint has not been reached. It is concerned with the formative process of getting there. Feedback is sometimes referred to as formative assessment.
2. Ende identifies for us that feedback should focus on all aspects of the student's developing professional competence, not just on the surface skills (psychomotor) but also on knowledge (cognitive) and feelings and attitudes (affectual behaviours).
3. Ende's point about clinical skills being more easily demonstrated (than described) underlines the importance of being able to observe the clinical process (providing the mirror). The clinical teacher has the major role in this but the professional has to learn to be his own reflector and therefore the student has to be helped towards ways of becoming self-critical, in preparation for IPR (Individual Performance Review) in their work.
4. Students are 'offered insights into', reminds us that as teachers we cannot *make* a student do something. What we need to ensure is that we have provided the enabling opportunities, for the identified goals to be reached.

5. In health care it is essential that the student is patient-oriented, so that the awareness that the outcomes of actions result in the delivery of care to clients should be held as central. It is a big step for the student to take, to centre on the needs of patients, instead of their own needs as learners.
6. Without feedback, as seen by the dancer in the mirror, good performance will not be recognized, while poor performance likewise will not be identified and adjusted. Clinical competence will only be achieved by a process of trial and error with patients as guinea pigs.

WHEN SHOULD FEEDBACK BE GIVEN?

Ideally feedback should be *immediate*. In the clinical situation this may not always be possible. Whether the student and clinician are in a college-based clinic or in a setting outside the college base, the principles of providing feedback remain the same. How and when feedback actually takes place will vary from one clinical setting to another and may also be delivered in somewhat different ways, across the professional groups.

In some professions it is relatively easy to provide immediate 'voice over' feedback by making suggestions to a student, while they are doing something with a patient. For example, in chiropody, orthoptics, physiotherapy and radiography it might be possible and acceptable to say to a student 'You might find it easier if . . .' or 'Mrs Jones might find it easier if you . . .' etc. Generally students feel supported by this kind of intervention, as usually they are aware when they are in a bit of a spot. This kind of approach fits in very well when something directly physical is being carried out. This is similar to the approach to teaching a procedure in gradual steps as outlined in Chapter 5. Cross (1992, pers. commun.) makes the important point that patients have to know that they are being treated by students and using 'voice over' feedback helps students to feel less pressurized into pretending to be more capable than they really are; they are then less anxious and more able to absorb the ongoing feedback. Nor do they lose face, as everyone is aware that they are a student.

In dietetics and speech language therapy it might not be as appropriate to use 'voice over' in this way because the clinical teacher's intervention cuts across the student–patient interchange, which is almost always taking place in these two fields as part of the clinical process. From observations and from discussions with students, it would appear that clinical teachers in dietetics and speech and language therapy might make more use of this kind of concurrent (voice-over) feedback. It is always as well to check with the student beforehand as to what they might feel about this type of intervention, or at least to alert them that you will use this approach. Generally students are happy for this to happen. Clinicians will need to judge if a student should or should not still be having concurrent feedback according to their stage of development. Obviously, when the safety of a patient is involved, the clinical teacher has to intervene.

If it is not possible to give feedback to a student during the treatment process, either because it is inappropriate or the clinician is not present, then ideally feedback should be given immediately after the treatment has finished. Approaches to fostering self-feedback, which is essential when the clinician is not present, will be explored below. When the clinical teacher has been able to observe the student for all or at least for part of the session (for example the clinician may be working with more than one student or more than one patient at a time) then feedback should take place as soon as the treatment has been completed. Because of the pressure of the case-load and the appointment system this may need to be fairly brief. It may therefore be advisable to timetable particular sessions for debriefing and feedback.

It might be possible to plan a programme for the duration of the placement: on an identified occasion, feedback will concentrate on work either of a specific case or on the student's progress with certain clinical competencies. Advance planning is likely to focus the student's attention and thus to accelerate learning. The following areas of generic skills relevant to all fields might form useful topics for feedback sessions:

- Case history taking
- Interaction with clients
- Counselling
- Team work

Where the student is supervised by a number of clinical teachers during the same placement period, for example on a block or sandwich placement, the feedback on generic skills will need to be informed by views gathered from all the members of the clinical teaching team. Following feedback the student should set goals, which should be made known to the clinical teaching team, so that everyone can help the student to achieve the agreed goals. The clinical teaching team will need to timetable into their own programme meeting times to review the student's progress. The frequency and timing of such meetings will need to be considered in the context of the stage of the course the student is at, as well as in relation to the clinical teacher's role in summative assessment, i.e. any formalized assessment at the end of an identified period.

In some professional groups, for example some physiotherapy and radiography placements, a monitoring/feedback session is timetabled at frequent, perhaps fortnightly, intervals. This is usually carried out by the clinical tutor appointed by the college to carry out regular teaching/supervisory sessions with students in clinic. This ongoing contact is not the same as occasional visits carried out by college tutors to students on placement. These visits will be considered later in this chapter.

When prompt feedback is not possible and the clinical teacher has observed the student working, it is advisable not to leave the student 'in the air'; this tends to increase the student's anxiety about their performance. It may even lead them to construe behaviours in the clinical teacher, as having some relationship to the clinical work they have just done. The student's own work will loom large in their mind, when in fact the clinician is concerned with many other pressing matters and is probably not even thinking about it. It may be helpful for the clinician to say, for example; 'I thought the session went quite well/well/very well. I'd like you to think about how it went so that we can talk about it later today/next week.' (Encouraging reflection time.) The provision of feedback on a regular and frequent basis helps to establish the student's own self-monitoring skills and ensures that problems do not mount up before they are tackled.

There are occasions when feedback needs to take a broader perspective than what has been done with a particular case or how skills are developing. From time to time, clinical teachers need to take stock to decide how a student is progressing with the aims set up for a particular setting, such as explored in Chapter 4. At other times it will be necessary to review how progress is being made towards the broader aims of the course and the overall aims of clinical competence. This kind of review serves to remind clinical teachers that arrangements and provisions may need to be set up for opportunities for the student to develop particular competencies. It might be helpful to make a list and divide this up into needs and goals (Box 7.1). For example, the student may need to improve their history taking skills with new patients, this would be listed as 2 in Box 7.1. Setting out needs and goals in this way defines more precisely what both the teacher and the student have to do.

Box 7.1 Setting needs and goals

NEEDS		GOALS	
1.	See more new patients.	1.	Improve interviewing skills, etc.
2.	See new patients who need a history taken.	2.	Improve history taking skills.
3.	Treat more CVA patients.		Increase my confidence in handling patients with hemiplegia.
4.	Attend clinical sessions with geriatrician.	4.	Improve my ability to talk to consultants.

HOW SHOULD FEEDBACK BE GIVEN?

'Let me know if you have any problems?' How many of us heard this when we were students in clinic? This kind of approach is not likely to meet any of the when, why or how criteria of giving feedback. This clinician is unlikely to be one who observes the student working, so that the clinician is not aware of the student's strengths and weaknesses. Initially, students do not have their own benchmarks for measuring their performance. They may well under-value their own fragile efforts and need to be reassured that they are doing all right. Other students may be realistically aware of their weaknesses and may be relieved that the clinician does not have a clear picture of what is going on.

When the clinician observes the student it is useful to keep some form of written record. This may be done as jottings to be fed back to the student verbally, in the post-session debriefing discussion, or it may be done in a more formal way. It may be helpful for the student and clinician to focus on just one aspect of competence or bring several together. The following could be selected for focus:

- Examination of patient
- Appropriateness of treatment
- Administration of treatment/procedure
- Ability to explain to patient
- Ability to motivate patient

It may be advisable to ask the student what they would like to attend to. This allows them to concentrate on their own concerns and make progress with them. Then, if necessary, the clinical teacher can lead on to address other areas of which the student seems unaware, or has not been ready to acknowledge and tackle.

Where a student has a number of problems it is not advisable to bring them all into focus at the same time, but to tackle each one in turn, thus engendering a feeling of progress and an ability to cope with difficulties. With some students it may indeed be hard to find strengths to reinforce. Students do have a tendency to remember the weak areas that have been identified in the feedback. It is, unfortunately, much easier for clinical teachers to be more explicit about what has not gone well. Constant efforts, therefore, need to be made to remember to tell the student about what *has* been done well. The provision of a written pro forma for the treatment session, which includes columns for positive and negative points, may help to remind the clinical teacher systematically to include the strengths.

After a feedback session has taken place it is important to give the student time to reflect on what has been said and to make a written record of what

Box 7.2 Pro forma for feedback on clinical session

PATIENTS NAME:			Date of session:
AIMS	METHODS/ EQUIPMENT		EVALUATION
		Patient's progress	Student's progress Strengths Weaknesses

AGREED GOALS FOR NEXT SESSION:

PATIENT:

STUDENT:

they understood the feedback to be about, including the objectives generated. This will ensure that a mismatch does not occur between the student's and the clinical teacher's perceptions. Mismatch appears to occur frequently. It may relate to the clinical teacher not giving clear feedback, possibly wrapping the point up to a degree where the student is unable to unravel what was intended. This may happen especially if the topic is perceived as sensitive. Mismatch may also occur when a student is not ready to accept the criticism.

At the beginning of a feedback session, the student should be given the first opportunity to talk about what went on. This helps to set the agenda for the student's main concerns and provides the clinical teacher with a view of the student's self-perception. Students express resentful feelings at being told about something which they themselves had been all too aware had not gone well. The preparation of a pro forma for both student and clinician use, suitable for (i) the particular profession and (ii) the particular setting or client, may be found useful in providing a more objective basis for feedback; a possible format is shown in Box 7.2. The use of this kind of pro forma enables the progress of the student to be closely related to the treatment aims and needs of an individual patient. In this way it is possible to say, for example, that a hemiplegic patient did not manage to walk well because the student's explanations or the physical help provided had been inappropriate or inadequate. Or that the patient did well because the student used a treatment competently, which was well targetted to the patient's needs. Review of the evaluation column over a period of time may reveal whether or not the student has persisting problems. After the feedback discussion with the clinical teacher the student should be ready to prepare further aims for the treatment of a patient and to draw up goals for their own development towards competence.

The pro forma in Box 7.3 takes a slightly different format. The clinician, who used this provided the following evaluation of its use. This illustrates the real problems and frustrations faced by a clinical teacher in working with a student who had a number of difficulties.

> Student and clinician tended to focus on the same areas of difficulty and in the session both found it hard to detail any successful areas. Student found it hard to extract specific points from the overall 'I felt out of control'. Discussed who was in control. Established that the mother was in control, but the student found it difficult to say why. Student observed the clinician the next day with particular reference to how control was established in the first 5 to 10 minutes, then the student found it easier to relate the feedback to her own session with the child.

Note how the clinician tries to resolve the problem by letting the student observe her handling the same clinical situation (note Ende's best demonstrated). The clinician commented that the student was very passive during the original feedback session and the clinical teacher commented that she felt 'pushed into the initiator, leader role, however hard I tried to share the initiative'.

The use of a pro forma has already been considered as a way of focusing on and recording the areas which need attention. The use of audio- and video-recording also provides a feedback mechanism. Feedback is most usually given through verbal interchange. In this context the points made earlier about the clinical teacher's direct or indirect style become extremely important.

Box 7.3 Alternative pro forma for feedback on clinical session. Carolyn Booth, Warwickshire Speech and Language Therapy Department

PATIENTS NAME:	CONDITION/DISORDER:
AREAS WHICH WENT WELL	AREAS OF DIFFICULTY
1. Control and management of session: 2. Timing, planning, organization: 3. Use of assessments: 4. General interaction:	
OBJECTIVES FOR THE STUDENT: OBJECTIVES FOR THE CLINICIAN:	

Pickering (1987) looks in detail at the communication process involved in the clinical teaching situation. She identifies ten behavioural skills which are associated with empathy, and which are of such importance in the provision of feedback. These skills are already likely to be within the clinical competence of health care professionals. It is therefore important to ensure that they are used in teaching students as well as in treating patients. The ten skills which Pickering lists are:

1. attending, acknowledging;
2. restating, paraphrasing;
3. reflecting;
4. interpreting;
5. summarizing, synthesis;
6. supportive questioning;
7. giving feedback;
8. supporting;
9. checking perceptions;
10. being quiet.

Although Pickering lists 'giving feedback' as a way of establishing empathy, in fact the behavioural skills she suggests would all need to be used in the feedback process. When negative criticism is included in the feedback it is essential that the clinical teacher leads the student on to seeing how the problems identified might be tackled.

At the end of placement it is important for feedback to be written down for the student. Some courses require that this is done in a formal way as part of the asssessment schedule. Present practice would suggest that when a report form is completed on a student's progress this should be seen and countersigned by the student. There should not be anything contained in the report of which the student is unaware. If there is, then it probably means that the process of providing feedback has not been effective. It is not helpful for a student to be made aware of a problem for the first time on returning to college, when the college tutor is reviewing clinical progress on the basis

Box 7.4 A students' own goals, following feedback

(a) *1st student*

1. Take a more active role in encouraging supervisors to push me more. I feel that I'm sometimes capable of doing more, but I fail to ask to be pushed, because I'm frightened of failing – if I was told to do something I would.
2. Do more administration in clinic.
3. To take initiative and not wait until somebody suggests doing something (i.e. confidence in dealing with someone in higher authority).
4. To think through every case for myself, and not just accept other therapists' opinions without reasoning for myself.
5. Make things interesting for children.
6. Develop my abilities to encourage patients.

(b) *2nd student*

1. Be myself.
2. Relate theory to practice.
3. Take more initiative and control of what is happening.
4. Think of myself more as a professional rather than a student.
5. Develop interaction skills with parents and relatives of patients.
6. Work on case history taking.
7. Get to grips with more assessment; know and understand what they can be used for – better selection of procedure.
8. Be more flexible – don't be scared to put my own ideas.

---

of the report received from the clinical teacher(s). Students are often heard to say: 'I didn't know that, why didn't they tell me before?'

If the student is not at the end of the course and there are further placements to be undertaken it is helpful if they prepare a list of objectives for the next placement, immediately following the placement feedback. Examples of objectives, written by students themselves, are shown in Box 7.4, a and b. It is interesting to study these objectives and try to decide how you would enable the student to realize them. You will notice that they tend to reveal something about the student as a whole.

WHO PROVIDES FEEDBACK TO THE STUDENT?

The clinical teacher

The prime person to provide feedback to the student is the clinical teacher who is working regularly with the student. The clinical teacher is a competent professional and is therefore a good judge of how a student is progressing. The clinical teacher, having observed the student working, is best able to judge whether the treatment and management of a patient is appropriate and effective for those patients who are the clinical teacher's responsibility. The judgment of a student's clinical progress is inevitably interwoven with the appropriateness of treatment; there is, therefore, a possible arena for conflict between clinical teachers and college tutors. Some monitoring arrangements adopted have a hidden agenda which is potentially devisive and may lead to what Jarvis (1983) describes as a rift between teachers and practitioners. The following practices are potentially devisive and should only be adopted after very careful consideration of the alternatives.

1. When students undertake clinical placements throughout the term, college-based clinical tutorials may be built into the college timetable. Even if these are meant to be mainly 'theoretical' it usually happens that the specific cases students are working with are used as illustrations in the discussions. No doubt these case illustrations provide valuable examples. However, this kind of discussion quite rightly and inevitably involves an evaluation of what is being done in clinic. It is difficult for students to leave this at an objective level. They have a tendency, no doubt, naively, to go back to the clinician and say 'X says I shouldn't or should be doing Y'.

2. In some fields, clinical tutors are appointed by the academic institution, to arrange student placements and monitor the student's progress on placements. These tutors are part of the institution in which the course is mounted. This may have a hidden message that clinical teachers are not fit to monitor the students' clinical progress and it needs someone

from the college base to do this. This may imply several things: college is more powerful; more academically respectable; knows all the answers; what is seen as practical (that which is done in clinic) is of a lower status than that which is theoretical (that which is taught in college). Staff appointed by the college are better judges than clinicans!?

Self-feedback

The final goal of the feedback provided by the clinical teacher should be to facilitate the student in becoming self-evaluative as part of professional competence. It therefore follows that students should gradually be expected to reflect more and more on their own work. The pro formas suggested earlier and shown in Boxes 7.2 and 7.3 are ways of encouraging students to become self-reliant in their feedback. Initially it may be necessary for the clinical teacher to steer the agenda for the feedback. For example, to say to the student after a session, 'I'd like you to tell me how you felt you managed the interview with Mr X.'

Where a pro forma has been used by both student and teacher, the teacher will have a clear picture of how insightful the student is becoming. When insight is developing well it may be possible to leave the student more on their own, giving them time to complete the pro forma for discussion later, or not discussing every pro forma but using the occasional 'dip sticks' to review progress.

It is useful, if possible, to introduce some other form of mirror. This can be done by the use of audio- or video-recording, if this is available. Recordings can only be used with the agreement of the patient concerned. Tape recorders are used routinely in speech and language therapy practice and could therefore be used for feedback to students. Dietitians could make valuable use of audio-recording as a learning aid for students. Some professions may use video-recordings in certain settings, such as child assessment centres. If these facilities are available they can be put to good use in student learning. All the professions could probably make use of audio-recording for students (and clinicians) to review some aspects, such as case history taking, explaining to and instructing patients, and advice and counselling. Listening and/or watching one's own performance deepens the understanding of what has taken place and enables enhancement and modification of the skills being used. If students make regular use of audio- and video-recording they will gradually become less anxious and learn to look on the recording as a help.

As a student progresses towards competence it may not be necessary to have feedback discussions on all areas of a treatment session. When the clinical teacher knows that a student is gradually becoming reliable it would be acceptable for students to signal when they feel the need for discussion about any problems that come up. This should of course include a grasp of the theoretical base on which the treatment is founded.

Feedback from peers

Some courses set the scene for peer group evaluation to take place early on, by arranging for students to observe other students who are at a more advanced stage of the course. As well as doing this in clinic, students can, if complicated timetables allow, be brought together for practical sessions. Some of the teaching methods outlined earlier, such as role play and patient simulation exercises can be usefully employed with students of different levels of experience. Watching other students is more easily arranged where there is a clinic within the college base.

Where more than one student attends a department there is an excellent opportunity for students to work in pairs. It may even be appropriate for them to treat a patient together; they can then take it in turns to be the 'clinician' or the observer. This enables students to give feedback to each other. They are usually found to be rigorous and open with each other in this task.

Where only one student is attending a clinic it is still important to try to set up an opportunity for peer evaluation. Perhaps arrangements could be made for students to visit each other in their clinical settings, where students are on long placements this should still be attempted. There may be other students elsewhere in the locality.

The use of peers as part of the feedback process may take some of the pressure off the very busy clinician, while ensuring that feedback continues. It may be particularly helpful in enabling the student to understand how they are progressing in the context of their peer group, rather than in the context of qualified experienced professionals.

Peer feedback is also important in laying down the concept that it is part of professional work to be observed and evaluated by one's own colleagues. This will help to prepare students for Individual Performance Review after qualification.

A student provided the following insights after visiting another student in her year group on clinical placement.

The visit took place with another student with whom the author felt she knew well and could relate to. This was most important because it was felt that each could be honest with the other about what they saw and offer the best constructive criticism. A number of advantages were immediately apparent after the day was over and they are listed below:

1. Opportunity to meet fellow student and compare notes and ideas.
2. Re-assurance that the kinds of activities you were doing were being done by others and were valid.
3. Collection of ideas enabled the collation of ideas and activities for the same problem.
4. Opportunity to see another student carrying out the same activity as you, used in a different, more or less successful way than you.
5. Observe patient types not seen much in your own placement.
6. Opportunity to see how other student (and therapist) handles something when things go wrong.
7. Opportunity to compare working situations and learn about different ways in which they operate.
8. Comparison of organisation of student placement, Allows one to come back and then relay the ideas to own supervisor about new ideas to improve the placement, if need be, and to talk about worries and problems you may have.

Patel, 1987, BSc Speech and Language Pathology and Therapeutics

Peer evaluation is used in the college setting, for example by getting students to read each others essays, or through the provision of a typed set of essays for students to criticize. These can be productive learning experiences. These learning methods are helpful in showing students the difference between standards. Although it is easier to set up opportunities for peer evaluation of written work in the college setting, in clinic, teachers may not do this because they may feel that students are not able to evaluate each other's clinical work. If opportunities have been provided for students to observe qualified practitioners, then they should be well-equipped to recognize good practice and from this to make comparisons.

There is evidence that students are able to evaluate their own work and, that their evaluations have a reasonable match with the evaluations of clinicians, although there are some differences in perceptions. Stackhouse and Furnham (1983) looked at the self-rating scales of students. To investigate the possible differences in perception of the clinical performance, comparisons were made between students', clinicians' and tutors' ratings of the students. To look at the predictive value of these ratings, correlations were run on the rating scores for each end of the year's practical and written examination results. Differences between raters did emerge and students were shown to be poor at predicting their final written and practical grades. However, an examination of students' rating scores compared with those of tutors and clinicians revealed that students tended to rate themselves almost invariably lower than did the college tutors and clinicians. We do not need to be concerned, therefore, as to whether students will evaluate themselves, but probably need to keep a watch that they are not too hard on themselves, although the researchers did wonder if the students were unwilling to produce high ratings because they saw themselves as learners. Clinicians provided the highest scores and college tutors midway between students and clinicians. This reminds us that, as clinical teachers, we need to be as objective in our work with students as we are in our work with patients.

The scales used by Stackhouse and Furnham rated eight elements of professional competence, from 0 (inadequate) to 6 (excellent), these were:

1. case history taking;
2. assessment of patients;
3. therapy;
4. social interaction and working relationships;
5. writing skills;
6. professional development;
7. present overall clinical competency;
8. potential overall clinical competency.

The authors stressed the importance of self-evaluation in encouraging students:

- Curiosity
- Discovery
- Personal satisfaction

They argued that if evaluation is done by clinicians and tutors alone students are locked into extrinsic-based learning, i.e. that which is done for examination purposes and attempting to please the supervisor/clinical teacher. Learning motivated in this way does not help to meet the need for qualified clinicians to be able to evaluate their own practice. Nor is it congruent with the needs and motivations of the adult learner. Every attempt must therefore be made to encourage students to appraise their own professional development.

The study by Stackhouse and Furnham raised some interesting points which need further consideration by both clinical teachers and college tutors. These were:

1. Do students set unrealistic goals for themselves?
2. Do students feel that they should quickly be at the same standard as their supervisors?
3. Do supervisors and college tutors allow for further learning through clinical placements and post-qualification experience which students have no concept of in the early stages of their training?

THE COLLEGE TUTOR VISIT AS PART OF THE FEEDBACK PROCESS

The study outlined above used college tutors in the research project. However the potential problems of using college tutors to evaluate students' clinical progress has already been raised. It has generally been the practice to make the main topic of a tutor visit, a student's work with individual patients; this seems to be true in all the health professions. Discussions between students, clinical teachers and college tutors suggest that in many fields the tutor visit may need to be reviewed. The following aspects of the visit need consideration:

- Purpose of the visit
- Timing frequency and length
- Content of the visit
- The role of the college tutor
- Problems identified by college tutors

Some purposes for the tutor visit are suggested in Box 7.5, these include purposes for all involved: student, clinician and visitor. Perhaps each participant should decide the purpose and see if these coincide.

Box 7.5 The purpose of the tutor visit

1. Nice for the student to see a familiar face.
2. The purpose should be flexible to meet individual needs.
3. For visiting tutor get to know clinicians and to support them.
4. Monitor placement.
5. Moderate standards.
6. Support student.
7. See how student operates in the setting, and how student is progressing.
8. See how the clinician and the student interact.
9. Consider the clinical teacher's assessment role.
10. Check programme to ensure that what the student is doing will meet the intended aims of the placement.
11. Check that needs are being catered for.
12. Provide opportunity for the student to discuss; personal, practical and academic matters.
13. Opportunity to update clinicians on: course requirements; continuing education opportunities.
14. Should be part of an ongoing process in the student's development, rather than purely assessment focused.
15. Provides the clinicians opportunity for personal contact with college tutors.
16. Explore links between theory and practice.
17. May provide opportunity for exchange of background information about student.
18. Help clinicians to explore their teaching role.
19. Facilitates feedback and goal setting.

Timing and frequency of the visit

It is essential that placements have ample notice of when a visit is to take place. Neville and French (1991) showed that students expressed dislike for unplanned visits by college tutors. Saxton and Ashworth (1990) also consider that unannounced visits are unacceptable. There is considerable value in early visits which establish that the student's needs are likely to be met. Early visits cannot be used for assessment and are therefore of special value in building the relationships between the clinical teacher, the visiting tutor and the student. Visiting students on placement is obviously costly in travel and staff time; there is little point in doing visits unless they are valuable to all concerned. Because of the unavoidable anxieties, sufficient time should be allowed for all participants to settle down and contribute in as relaxed and honest a way as possible. It does not help if the clinician and student feel that the visitor is having to rush off. If major problems arise it is essential that the visitor 'hangs in' until some acceptable way forward is found. Some points about timing and frequency are summarized in Box 7.6.

Box 7.6 Timing and frequency of the visit

---
1. If visits are not related to assessment they can be brought earlier. Such timing may allow other purposes to become more central.
2. Need for more visits to new clinical teachers/placements.
3. Timing should relate to individual student needs.
4. Clinicians should be given plenty of warning of tutor visit.
5. Timing and purpose are closely related.
6. Sufficient time should be allowed to enable all participants to settle down and contribute in as honest and relaxed a way as possible. With opportunity to raise issues which they see as important.

The content of the visit

If the view is adopted that the clinical teacher is, firstly experienced as a judge and secondly, is the person responsible for the treatment of the patients, the student is working with, then this frees the visit time for the exploration of other issues. For example establishing that the expectations of the clinical teacher match those of the college tutor, at the given stage of the course, or of exploring methods of teaching and learning. Some ideas on the content of the visit are listed in Box 7.7.

Box 7.7 Content of the tutor visit

---

1. Should the student be seen with clients/patients;
   Is this representative of the student's work?
   Could the student present a case study, instead of the actual case?
2. College tutor needs to be a negotiator.
3. Need for opportunity for more feedback from the student.
4. Visits that focus on theory may be very anxiety provoking.
5. Counselling/discussion most helpful.
7. Need time to air views, have feedback, input of theory, match college/clinic expectations.
8. Need to focus on student aims and their realization.
9. Should the tutor: see the student alone; see the clinician without the student?
10. Is it possible for the tutor to meet a number of clinicians if the student is being supervised by several clinical teachers.
11. Discussing and exploring potential range of experiences.
12. Exploring teaching methods appropriate to the workplace.
13. All participants should have a say in setting the agenda for the visit.

The role of the college tutor in the visit

All those involved in the visit need to understand their particular role. The role of the visitor should have been explored by the course team. Where a number of staff are involved in visiting students it is essential that aims and content are agreed by the group. Relevant points are listed in Box 7.8.

Some professional groups appear to have clearly defined aims for tutor visits. An example from physiotherapy lists suggestions that tutors visiting placements should check that 'clinical educators' (clinical teachers), can demonstrate:

1. Provision of a suitable learning environment for the student.
2. Knowledge of the student's entry behaviour.
3. Qualities of a teacher likely to assist or promote the success of student learning.
4. Application of some strategies and tactics in teaching and student learning.
5. Skills in the use of questioning to elicit appropriate level of intellectual activity on the part of the student.
6. Ability to demonstrate a skill to a student and or to correct a student's inappropriate application of the same to a patient.
7. An understanding of the purpose of student assessment.
8. Assessment of a student's ability to base practice on theoretical insights and to use practice to test theory.

Box 7.8 The role of the college tutor in visiting students on placement

> 1. Provide a link between course and placement agency. Establish and maintain liason.
> 2. Provide and maintain a link between course and student.
> 3. To stimulate optimum conditions for learning.
> 4. Ensure that all reach an agreed understanding of the stage the student has reached.
> 5. Help to identify future goals.
> 6. Obtain feedback about current college teaching, as reflected in the student's knowledge, approaches, etc.
> 7. Provide opportunity for discussion of teaching/learning processes.
> 8. Clarify specific aspects of philosophy and content of a course.
>
> TUTOR'S VISITS ARE NOT FOUND TO BE HELPFUL
> IF:
>
> 1. the visit is billed as an assessment when it is not;
> 2. there is over-emphasis on individual cases;
> 3. clinicians are not prepared to be open about student, course, tutor, etc.;
> 4. the visit is seen as an opportunity to give the student feedback which has not been given before;
> 5. if clinicians working with the student have not been able to free time for discussion with the student and tutor, during the visit;
> 6. the student is put on show with a 'good' or 'interesting' patient.

9. Ability to determine progress of the student at appropriate intervals during clinical experience.
10. Awareness of the problems of subjectivity in student assessment.

Saxton and Ashworth (1990) provide a very fruitful discussion on the topic of tutor visits to placements. Their recommendations on the nature and content of the visits and the role of the visiting tutor are based on a study of the observations of a large number of visits. Although the study was concerned with sandwich placements not in health settings, they raise remarkably similar concerns to our own. They discuss the importance of timing and the amount of time the tutor spends on a visit. They stress the importance of involving all the participants (supervisor, student and visiting tutor) in contributing to the agenda. They describe a scenario where the visitor felt that the visit had gone well but the student and the supervisor were left feeling very frustrated, as they had not been given the chance to address their concerns; the participants here all had a different view of the visit. This highlights the need for great sensitivity on the part of the visiting tutor. Saxton and Ashworth emphasize the tremendous value of placement experience on student learning and the consequent importance of visits:

> Placement is an important, some might argue potentially the most important, aspect of a course and visits should never be treated as a side issue or a chore. Therefore staff and the institution should place proper value on the visits and allocate sufficient time, staff and financial resources to them.

A colleague with considerable experience both as a clinician, a clinical teacher and college tutor provided the following valuable insights into the tutor visit:

1. 'Success' of a visit should not be equated with how well the student is/is said/is thought to be progressing.
2. When there are problems, that is when the greatest demand is put on the tutor's teaching/communication skills. I count a visit as successful if I have been able to confront problems, communicate them to the student and or supervisors and to facilitate **mutual decision-making**. I see myself as the one with responsibility here.
3. If no serious problems present then it is still important to identify future aims jointly. This can be delicate, as college tutor's behaviour in this instance can be interpreted as 'nit-picking' or threatening. Success equals conveying the necessity for an active approach to learning (for the student), and teaching (for the supervisor), without making unrealistic demands or antagonising anyone.
4. Social elements in a visit, e.g. working lunch at pub or canteen can be very valuable in meeting the team and exploring each other's strengths and interests in the work setting.
5. Professional attitudes emerge which are of relevance to how the student is being socialised into the profession.
6. Seeing a student in a clinical session gives the opportunity for several areas to be addressed: Success equals (i) if the general issue of giving feedback can be discussed around the concrete features emerging from the session. If student and clinician see this as a central part of the learning processs; (ii) if the student's self-evaluation is promoted in some way; (iii) if the student is enable to relate technical performance to theoretical bases.
7. Be aware that clinicians' perceptions of the visit may be different from the tutor's (and the student's!)
8. I see the particular role for the tutor as the ability to abstract from the concrete elements of the placement, as seen on the day of the visit,

and attribute these abstractions to a generalised educational philosophy/methodology. The need to extract meaning from experience and to organise and classify out of the vast complexity of clinical/-professional education.

SUCCESS equals when I have been able to make the above kinds of interpretations for myself and perhaps to express them verbally at points in the student/clinician/tutor interchange.

Rowan, 1987

In making these points it is in no way being suggested that the college should not have a monitoring role in the student's progress on placement. Obviously college has a major responsibility for the students and their overall progress. However, there are a number of ways that this responsibility may be fulfilled.

Closely related to this is the issue of the student's summative evaluation (final assessment). The role of the clinical teacher, the college tutor and the role of the external examiner in relation to clinical assessment will be considered in the next chapter.

Box 7.9 Summary of reasons for giving feedback

---

1. To encourage the student to reflect on the work they are doing.
2. To lead the student towards independent practice, which includes the evaluation of practice.
3. To build the student's competence, and to ensure that the full range of professional competencies are laid down.
4. To build the student's confidence in their own skills.
5. To provide opportunity for the student to try out knowledge in the reality of practice.
6. To identify strengths and weaknesses.
7. To identify precisely what needs to be worked on, in order to facilitate behavioural change.
8. To ascertain if there are discrepancies between the clinician and student's expectations and perceptions.
9. To ensure that students are given help and guidance in areas where they feel a need.
10. To ensure that students do not miss out because they feel unable to ask for feedback. Clinicians have the responsibility to be the initiators here.
11. To help students to arrive at a complete view of the professional role as well as to attend to the detail within it.

From the discussions in the above sections it is hoped that the need for feedback in assisting the student's learning is now clear. It is probably the most important teaching method available to the clinical teacher. The reasons for giving feedback are summarized in Box 7.9.

FEEDBACK TO THE COURSE, THE PLACEMENT AND THE CLINICAL TEACHERS

It is the responsibility of the institution providing the course to ensure that the work experience elements of the course are productive learning experiences for the student. Generally this challenging, and no doubt stressful job is fulfilled by the clinical teachers. As part of the complete cycle of monitoring and evaluation, students need to provide feedback to course managers on their work experience. The following examples of difficulties faced were provided by students. They were collected anonymously from a student group.

1. 'Clinician too dominant: sat in with me every session. Told me when to talk to teachers and what to say. I found the situation very humiliating – it also wasn't allowing me to develop my own clinical skills and to make decisions.'
2. 'Difficulties of policy plans in the District and the advice college give, e.g. school visits, are emphasized in college, yet the districts may have a policy which does not allow for visiting a child in school.'
3. 'Student is seeing a patient for the first time. No one else has seen the patient and it is obvious from the interview that the patient does not require and in fact does not want therapy. In the middle of the interview the clinician joins the student, who explains to the clinician about the patient. The clinician then steps in and discharges the patient. Afterwards the student is reprimanded for not having made this decision.'
4. 'I saw a very young child with behaviour problems, with both the mother and the therapist observing me.'
5. 'In week one of my placement the clinician asked me to take an assessment five minutes before the client arrived.'
6. 'I was not given feedback about my personal performance until my tutor's visit – then they told me and my tutor at the same time. I should have made it clear at the time that I preferred them to tell me about my performance, so that I could adjust accordingly.'
7. 'The clinician felt that the patients were her exclusive property and that no intervention by the student should be undertaken without the clinician being present. Certainly no management decisions should be made. The role of the student was as a general helper, passive learner, no 'hands on' contact.'
8. 'The therapist had set ways of dealing with certain disorders and was not amenable to new ideas that the student wanted to try.'

No doubt if clinicians listed their problems as clinical teachers they might well come up with a list which provides almost the opposite perceptions of similar scenarios. There is obviously the potential for different perceptions. Each of the problems identified is worth separate analysis, but there are a number of factors which are worth general comment. In some instances perhaps lines of accountability and responsibility could have been made clearer to the student. Other examples suggest personality factors may be operating, either in the student or the clinical teacher. Sometimes students may need to be more assertive and request the opportunity to observe the clinician first of all in an area in which the student does not feel confident (e.g. Point 4 above). In some of the examples there is clearly a need for greater dialogue between the college and the placement. In others it seems likely that the clinician needs to take time to consider the clinical teaching role. However most of the problems can be traced to the interpersonal relationship and communication between the student and the clinician.

Knowledge of these problems by course managers does raise the difficult question of how feedback might best be provided for the clinical teachers. This is a very sensitive area and therefore one which is unfortunately usually avoided. As yet I have not come across a course which feels it can handle this matter satisfactorily.

Some placements give students the opportunity to give feedback by providing an appropriate section in the information pack. Examples of feedback pro forma, used by three different professional groups, can be seen in Boxes 7.10, 11 and 12. They would all help to provide valuable information to the receiving placement. Clinical teachers who offer students opportunities to give this kind of feedback are without doubt receptive in their work with students, viewing

Box 7.10 Feedback on placement: Chiropody. Adapted from Portsmouth and South East Hampshire Health Authority

---

Short questionnaire to include the following:

1. Did you consider that the time spent on this placement was of value?
2. Did you receive enough practice?
3. Did you get enough support from the clinician in charge?
4. Do you generally enjoy this area of clinical practice?
5. Did you feel part of the team?
6. Was the student pack of interest/help to you?
7. Do you have any suggestions for improving the student pack?
8. Did you make use of the observation sheet?
9. Did you enjoy your time on this placement?

Box 7.11 Feedback on placement: Speech and Language Therapy Department. Adapted from Portsmouth and South East Hampshire Health Authority

---

1. Were you given enough information to benefit fully from your placement?
   (a) on environment, transport, etc.
   (b) information on resources, equipment, etc.
   (c) the structure of the department, staff, etc.
   (d) expertise within the department.
   (e) expertise outside the department.
2. Did the clinical experience match your needs and expectations?
   (a) patients: number, variety and complexity?
   (b) range of clinics.
   (c) appropriateness of discussion?
3. Did the clinicians have sufficient knowledge of your needs early on in the placement?
   If not can you think of any preparation we might make for the future?
4. Can you offer any suggestions to other students to benefit from while working here?

Box 7.12 Feedback on placement: orthoptics. Adapted from Feedback Form on Clinical Experience, School of Orthoptics, Leeds

---

TICK UNDER THE APPROPRIATE COLUMN YOUR VIEWS ON THE FOLLOWING STATEMENTS.

Box 1 VERY GOOD   Box 2 SATISFACTORY   Box 3 UNSATISFACTORY

	1	2	3
1. The range of patients seen was			
2. The time allowed for each patient examination was			
3. The time for discussion of the patient was			
4. The value to your professional development was			
5. The clarity of explanation of management was			
6. The ability to feel part of the department was			
7. The preparation of the patient, so that he/she knew that they were being seen by a student was			
8. The availability of testing equipment was			
9. The access to help when needed was			
10. The occurrence of supervision, when not requested by the student was			

---

their role as a learning experience and showing eagerness to be effective teachers. Receiving agencies which demonstrate this kind of approach to the job of working with students are not likely to be a cause of concern to the institution placing the student. Eliciting feedback from the student by the host placement is much the best way of providing feedback. It can become a problem if matters have to be taken up by the institution because the placement has not tried to elicit feedback for themselves.

Inevitably there will be some occasions when feedback from student and visiting tutors indicate that all is not well and that a particular setting may not be constructive in student learning. When the course team is aware that there is a problem and that action needs to be taken it is still very difficult to decide how this should be done. If difficulties relate to one specific clinical teacher it might be advisable for the course tutor to have an informal word with the head of department/unit/service. Some posts in health care carry a clinical teaching responsibility as part of the job description, there is therefore a responsibility for the health authorities to provide continuing education opportunities in the area of clinical teaching, as well as for the institution placing the students to offer educational opportunities to clinical teachers, such as short courses, workshops, and briefing sessions. The designation of one member of staff in a department as having special responsibility in clinical teaching, may help to deal with the problems of providing feedback and facilitate a clear channel of communication between the course and the service.

Short courses, briefing sessions, etc., provide a medium for general feedback to clinical teachers as well as opportunities for less experienced clinicians to meet the more experienced. It also provides a forum for clinical teachers to feed in views and air their problems with the course team. Problems frequently reported by clinical teachers are: not wanting to overload the student or not giving them enough to do; time for the student always grabbed at the end of the day; limited information beforehand on what the student has done or on what the student wants to do on placement and the difficulties in giving negative feedback.

Mechanisms must be found to give feedback to the course on such matters as:

1. How well students have been prepared for the placement experience.
2. The adequacy of the information provided by the course.
3. The value and conduct of tutor visits.
4. The assessment process.

Short courses can be of particular value when offered on a multidisciplinary basis, while workshops and briefing sessions are most likely to have a single professional or course focus. The latter are particularly useful in the process of course evaluation and development.

Recently qualified clinicians should, where possible, be included in all educational events related to clinical teaching as they can provide unique insights from their own recent experiences as students, while at the same time becoming prepared for their future role as clinical teachers.

SUPPORT NETWORKS

Every opportunity should be found to support clinicians in their role as clinical teachers, which in turn will be of benefit to students. A number of networks should be explored.

- Student   with College tutor
- Student   with Clinical teacher/tutor
- Student   with Peers
                                    – in own field
                                    – in other fields
- Clinical teacher with College tutor
- Clinical teacher with Other clinical teachers
                                    – in own department
                                    – set up by course
- Clinical teacher with Colleagues in department
                                Manager of service
- Clinical teacher with Colleagues in other settings
- Clinical teacher with Clinical teachers in other fields

FOLLOW-UP ACTIVITIES

1. Review when you provide feedback to students. Consider whether this meets students needs. It might be helpful to discuss this with the students.
2. Make a list of generic skills, which could be the subject of feedback in your own professional sphere.
3. Consider if there are opportunities where you might use 'voice over' feedback with students. Assess whether you make appropriate use of these. Ask students what they might consider to be helpful.
4. Design a feedback pro forma which could be used in your own setting. Try it out and see how it influences your feedback session with a student.
5. Consider ways of encouraging students to use peer feedback in your clinical setting.
6. Taking the example of one student, list out the forms of feedback which have been used in helping his/her development.

7. If you do not already do so, encourage the student to make a brief written summary of a feedback session, for their personal use. Get them to share with you the goals it generated.
8. Think about the way the tutor visits are undertaken for the students in your clinics. Do the visits meet the students needs and your needs as a clinical teacher?
9. Examine the pro formas in Boxes 7.10, 7.11 and 7.12. From these examples design a pro forma suitable for use by students attending your clinical setting.

REFERENCES

Argyris, C. and Schon, D. (1974) *Theory in Practice: increasing Professional Effectiveness*, Jossey Bass, San Francisco.

Ende, J. (1983) Feedback in Clinical Medical Education. *Journal of American Medical Association*, 12 August, **250**, 6, 777–81.

Jarvis, P. (1983) *Professional Education*, Croom Helm, London.

Neville, S. and French, S. (1991) Clinical Education: Students' and Clinical Tutors' Views. *Physiotherapy*, **17**, no. 5, 351–4.

Pickering, M. (1987) Interpersonal Communication and the Supervisory Process, in Crago, M. and Pickering, M. (eds) *Supervision in Communication Disorders*, College Hill Publications, Boston.

Saxton, J. and Ashworth, P. (1990) Sandwich Degree Placements and Visiting Tutors. *Journal of Further and Higher Education*, **14**, no. 1, 31–50.

Stackhouse, J. and Furnham, A. (1983). A student-centred Approach to the evaluation of clinical skills. *British Journal of Disorders of Communication*, **18**, no. 3, 171–9.

Warrender, F. (1990) Clinical Practice: A Student Centred Learning Package. *British Journal of Occupational Therapy*, **53**, no. 6, 233–8.

8

The assessment of professional competence

INTRODUCTION

The assessment of competence in all the fields with which we are concerned is a very complex area and can only be addressed at an introductory level in one chapter in a book of this nature, Heron (1988) suggests that there are four parts to the process of assessment: what to assess, which criteria to use, how to apply the criteria and how to do the assessment itself. These four points will be addressed in the discussion which follows.

This chapter uses the term 'professional competence', rather than 'clinical competence' in order to reflect the wide range of work activities in which health professionals are engaged. This orientation reminds us that, in deciding what to assess at the end of a course, we should not only attend to the patient-focused elements of the job but also to the assessment of such aspects as working with colleagues, self-management, management of others, ability to record accurately, communication with others in the health team, awareness of ethical standards, responsibility, confidentiality, etc., all essential aspects of the work of the professional.

It is best if the final (summative) assessment of the student in their 'practical' work, is not thought of as something separate from what has gone on before in the student's development. It follows on from the feedback process (formative assessment), which has continued throughout a student's course, and which was discussed in Chapter 7. Saxton and Ashworth (1990) also see summative assessment as developing naturally from the formative assessment process. The student's self-assessment, together with assessment by clinical teachers and college tutors, preceded by and followed by setting objectives and working towards achieving them, again receiving feedback and making further progress, is all part of the ongoing process of continuous assessment.

This has a formative role in preparing students for their chosen professional field. However, at some specified point, at the end of a placement or the whole course, a mark or grade has to be assigned to the standard reached. Along with this, a decision is made as to whether or not the individual is safe to proceed to the next stage or, more importantly, to enter professional practice.

Clinicians who are new to clinical teaching are understandably concerned about their ability to carry out assessment and therefore their responsibility in relation to the student's final assessment. Clinical teachers from all fields express their concern at being asked to be involved, particularly in the final summative assessment of students. Cross (in press) describes the running of a needs analysis workshop for clinical teachers in physiotherapy. She got the clinical teachers to identify 'incidents or situations, related to student learning, which they remembered as causing them discomfiture, anxiety or difficulty', and then to list questions which were raised by the incidents. A number of the questions generated were related to formative and summative assessment:

- How clinicians cope with guilt feelings about students?
- Do all clinicians fail students when they think they should?
- How can we help students to grasp the concept of constructive criticism and involve them in the process more?

Clinical teachers may not be experienced assessors of students, although they are obviously experienced at assessing patients. They are experienced professionals, well able to recognize acceptable levels of professional practice in others. Of course, assessment becomes somewhat easier when there has been opportunity to work with a number of different students and therefore to compare standards across students completing a course. On the occasions when it is necessary, it is not easy to reach a decision to fail a student. This is never easy, either for the experienced or inexperienced. Problems related to failing students will be discussed further later in the chapter.

THE NEWLY QUALIFIED PROFESSIONAL

A good place to start thinking about the assessment of competence is for clinical teachers to ask themselves what they would expect of a newly qualified person coming to work in their department. Apart from a few weeks' vacation there is usually nothing between this stage and when the same individual qualified a few weeks earlier. We cannot of course compare a new practitioner's fragile competence even with that of someone with a few months experience, but the elements must be clearly established in the newly qualified. Caney (1983) describes this as 'operational competence' where the new professional has achieved satisfactory, although partial, integration of the three elements of knowledge, skills and attitudes. You may now like to look at the first follow-up activity for this chapter, on p. 196 and do it now.

What we expect from the newly qualified

Professionals do not seem to have any problem about identifying the expectations they have of a newly qualified person joining their department. Lists of such expectations generated through discussion with professional groups can be found in Boxes 8.1, 8.2 and 8.3.

It is interesting to note that apart from the reference to biomechanical knowledge and anaesthesia in chiropody, very few of these expectations are about the specific knowledge-base of the field. Is there a presumption that this will obviously be present and will have been assessed by various methods? References are made to knowledge more broadly: 'Be safe – knowledge of basic techniques'. 'Have good knowledge and be able to update others'. Or is it because it is so important and central that we don't even remember to mention it? Hopefully it is not that we do not see it as being very important as part of professional competence!

Box 8.1 Orthoptists' expectations of a new entrant

Ability to:
1. diagnose accurately;
2. make some decisions;
3. recognize own limitations;
4. make day-to-day decisions on work-load;
5. be able to write full, appropriate and accurate reports;
6. communicate with patients and staff;
7. conduct themselves in a clinical situation;
8. be adaptable.

Box 8.2 Physiotherapists' expectations of a new entrant

1. Basic knowledge of anatomy and physiology and the patient's condition.
2. Ability to set and carry out treatment plan.
3. Ability to be *safe* – knowledge of basic techniques (under supervision).
4. Knowledge of limitations.
5. Ability to communicate and be aware of their role within the team.
6. Ability to review and to evaluate treatment.

Box 8.3 Speech and Language Therapists' expectations of a new entrant

Ability to:

1. manage time;
2. organize case-load;
3. prioritize case-load;
4. produce professional reports and record information;
5. form good working relationships;
6. interview, assess, plan treatment;
7. ask for help in long-term planning;
8. appear competent;
9. respect rules (unspoken);
10. have a good knowledge-base and be able to update others;
11. have ideas of where they want to go in their career;
12. respect boundaries and rules of establishment;
13. use initiative;
14. be confidential.

WHAT IS TO BE ASSESSED?

It is up to each course and to each field as a whole to identify which competencies are essential requirements for an individual to be judged as competent to enter practice. It is always difficult to reach a consensus in deciding what should be included. Although it is essential that all three elements of knowledge, skills and attitudes are included. Students are likely to have their knowledge quite thoroughly assessed through college-based assessments, such as in essays and unseen written examinations. Whether these are satisfactory ways of assessing knowledge is another matter.

It is possible for some students to have an adequate or even good knowledge-base, but not to have integrated it with the other elements and therefore to be poor at applying their knowledge to the particular problems of patients in clinical practice. You will remember the Schwab (1969, 1971) definitions we looked at in Chapter 1. The course assessment diet should therefore also include assessments which demonstrate a cognitive grasp of how to apply general knowledge to particular problems met on the job. Such methods as the compilation of log books, which must include an evaluative component (as discussed in Chapter 2), case histories, case studies (see also p. 191 below), which help to demonstrate if the student has an intellectual grasp of whether what is going on clinically, are useful. We need to attend to the two ends of the theory–practice continuum. Most importantly the assessment of clinical competence, either through continuous assessment or some form of practical examination, must include the knowledge element of competence.

As discussed earlier it is not possible to be competent in practice unless practice includes what is going on in the head of the practitioner, otherwise we might just be preparing technicians who can skillfully carry out prescribed procedures. Some of the main areas of knowledge are suggested in Box 8.4.

Box 8.4 The main areas of knowledge which need to be included in the assessment of clinical competence

---

Each of these headings could be divided into subheadings appropriate to a given field.
1. Knowledge of the range of conditions, which can normally be met with in the field.
2. Knowledge of observational and descriptive procedures, in order to identify and analyse the nature of the disorder.
3. Understanding the criteria for selection of assessment/measurement procedures.
4. Competence in the identification of a disorder, and related causal and maintaining factors.
5. Knowledge necessary to formulate management/treatment plan, to select and implement appropriate management/treatment.
6. Ability to evaluate the efficacy of the management/treatment.

Assessing skills is probably the easiest element of competence to assess because it is visible on the surface and can be related to specific behavioural objectives. Skills relating to assessment, diagnosis and treatment all need to be assessed, and it is these which have to rest securely on a knowledge base. Box 8.5 provides examples of the types of general skills to be assessed in a range of fields.

We need to ensure that assessment of competence not only includes knowledge and skills but perhaps most important of all, that **attitude** is included. This is the most difficult element to assess, so the easiest route is to ignore it as part of the assessment, especially at the summative stage and hope and presume that it is present. Others may have done the same earlier on in the student's course, or presume that appropriate attitudes will develop in future. So it may be possible to find that there are practitioners in our own field who we would judge as not having an appropriate professional attitude. One positive finding is that health professionals are not averse to assessing practice, apparently unlike some other fields. Chatterton *et al.* (1988), in business and engineering degrees, found a reluctance to assess anything which

Box 8.5 The main areas of skills which need to be included in the assessment of clinical competence

---

Each of these headings could be broken down into detail appropriate to a given field.

Ability to:

1. carry out all procedures at the maximum safety levels, for the physical and psychological well being of the patient/client;
2. relate effectively and appropriately, to clients/patients and others in the working situation;
3. carry out appropriately selected assessment/measurement procedures, efficiently and effectively;
4. carry out appropriately and efficiently treatment procedures;
5. carry out procedures with due sensitivity to client/patient;
6. adjust the execution of treatment procedures in the light of any unexpected responses, reactions, etc.;
7. allocate time appropriately, and prepare in advance for the treatment of patients;
8. prepare materials and equipment safely and appropriately;
9. write notes accurately on treatment given and patient response.

Box 8.6 Examples of attitudes to be included in the assessment of clinical competence

---

1. A positive and responsible attitude to the working situation.
2. Willingness to evaluate own work.
3. Ability to obtain and respond to advice from colleagues.
4. Ability to maintain appropriate objectivity in all matters concerning the welfare of clients/patients.
5. Independent attitude to continuing education, showing a willingness to update knowledge and skills.
6. Respect for patients/clients, providing privacy, etc.
7. Integrity, loyality and dependability.
8. Ability to take full responsibility for own decisions and actions.

---

was viewed as being outside the cognitive domain. Box 8.6 lists some of the attitudinal elements of competence, which have been included in the assessment of some health care fields.

Health professions have taken a great deal of trouble in trying to reach an agreement on what constitutes competence. Reaching a consensus is sometimes done through the Delphi Method (Helmer, 1964). This procedure first generates a list of competencies from various sources. These are then gradually refined through consultation and feedback from an identified panel of 'experts' in the field, until a consensus is reached. There is, however, still a considerable step between agreeing what the competencies are which should be judged and deciding what form of assessment is to be used and then actually judging the competencies agreed.

WHAT FORM DOES THE ASSESSMENT OF
PROFESSIONAL COMPETENCE TAKE?

There are a number of different assessment formats to be found in courses for health professionals. Clinical teachers will need to decide if the format they are involved with falls into one of those listed below, or if they use some other form. Some possible formats are:

1.   continuous assessment only;
2.   continuous assessment plus final practical examination;
3.   final examination only:
     (a) on placement,
     (b) back in college;
4.   final examination plus some form of oral or written examination:
     (a) oral examination on cases,
     (b) log book,
     (c) diary,
     (d) project
     (e) case studies.

For each of these it is necessary for the clinical teacher to know his/her role in the assessment processes. We will consider each format in turn.

Continuous assessment only

This would seem to be a procedure which will involve the clinical teacher (in clinics away from the college-base), more than any other method of assessment. It is a good method because it can be the least invasive in relation to the day-to-day ongoing work of the student. Nevertheless, it is recognized that sometimes it is difficult for the clinical teacher to make objective judgements about the student because of the nature and continuity of the relationship between them and the many different roles the clinical teacher has to fulfill (Cox, 1988). It may be helpful for clinicians to think of it as similar to the evaluation to be made of a patient's progress, which also has to be objective. It is possible, unfortunately, for the student to feel that they are under the continuous pressure of close scrutiny.

Collaborative assessment

The other consideration is whether or not the student should be involved in the assessment. There is some evidence that clinical teachers tend to be generous in their judgement of student standards while, interestingly, students assessing themselves tend to be too harsh. Tutors from courses tend to stand somewhere in the middle (Stackhouse and Furnham, 1983). We looked at this study before in relation to feedback in Chapter 7. The findings of this study of speech and language therapy students also has some interesting implications about who should be involved in the assessment of students. The ideal would seem to be contributions from the triad of student, clinical teacher and college tutor to achieve a consensus. The traditional model, where teaching staff carry out the assessment, is inappropriate to experiential learning; the use of college tutors alone is inappropriate. Furthermore, the clinical teacher's facilitative role makes their assessment role a difficult one; collaborative assessment, involving all parties concerned, is therefore essential.

Some problems which emerged from the Stackhouse and Furnham (1983) study were:

1. Students may set unrealistic goals for themselves? Especially as they feel they should quickly be at the same level as their clinical teachers/ supervisors.
2. Clinical teachers and college tutors allow for further learning, which students have no concepts of in the early stages of their training.
3. Students may be unwilling to present higher ratings of themselves because they see themselves in the learner role.

It also became clear that when only clinical teachers and college tutors were involved in the assessment, that students' motivations were purely extrinsic – to pass the examinations and please the clinical teacher. If self-evaluation was included, however, curiosity, discovery and self-satisfaction were encouraged.

Self-evaluation is an essential element in performance review of professional work (IPR), and it is therefore important to lay down the concepts of self-evaluation during the learning phase. This is also in accord with the needs of adult learners and developing student autonomy, discussed earlier. Heron (1988) stresses that the 'unilateral control of students by staff (in assessment) generates the wrong set of motivation in students'. He also claims that where educational systems are authoritarian they are only able to focus on intellectual and technical competence. The other elements, such as personal development, interpersonal skills and feelings, tend to be excluded from the curriculum and presumably the assessment process. Heron makes a strong case for collaborative assessment.

The differences in judgement between students and others can also be found outside the health area. Chatterton *et al.* (1988) in their study of business students say; 'there is a common view held among tutors that the companies assess students too generously (as compared to the student's self-assessment which is too harsh' (p. 160). This severity of students in their self-assessment has also been noted in research by the Council for National Academic Awards (1989).

Everyone involved needs help in carrying out assessments. There is a need for ongoing discussion between the course, the clinical teachers and the students. Opportunities should be provided to support participants in their assessment responsibilities, through attention to the topic in courses for clinical teachers, and in setting up a joint forum for clinicians, students and college tutors, when assessment criteria should be agreed and methods discussed. It is particularly important to support clinical teachers and the institutions receiving students on placements through providing courses. This will upgrade the standard of teaching and supervision, and help to achieve some parity of standard across placements. This is of extreme importance in relation to assessment because students are judged as if they have had the same placement experiences, which of course they have not.

Continuous assessment plus final practical examination

In addition to the student being assessed by the clinical teacher(s), who is (are) responsible for completing a report, another practical assessment (usually a one-off examination) is sometimes carried out as well. This is done either in the clinic, where the student is placed, or in a college-based clinic. If this is the format there are some points to consider. First, how are the marks or grades weighted between the continuous assessment and the examination element? Is the grade added, in some way, to the result of the continuous assessment, or doesn't the continuous assessment carry a mark towards the result of the course overall? Secondly, what does the implementation of the college examination suggest about the status and competence of the clinical teachers in relation to their ability to assess the student. The relative weighting may reveal the views underlying this. It would seem to be a format where there are unfortunate messages about the status of clinical teachers. The approach is devisive and not conducive to fostering a 'community of learning', where decisions are shared. Is it to do with the course's need to 'control' what is going on, the authoritarian institution referred to by Heron (1988)? It may arise from pressure from professional bodies or statutory bodies which govern registration. It could, however, be because 'we've always done it like that' and it is locked into the history of the profession or the course.

Final examination only on placement

In this format the student is examined on the placement by the visiting college tutor. In this instance the role of the clinical teacher is of particular interest. What is their role? Do they carry out the assessment jointly with the tutor (in which case two qualified people observe the student) and how is this organized? What can the clinical teacher learn about the student's work on this occasion which is not already known? Or does the tutor 'examine' the student alone and then discuss the findings with the clinical teacher and the grade/mark is arrived at by joint discussion? Or does the tutor make a unilateral assessment and decision? Are there still problems about status here? Furthermore, is the student involved in any way in reaching the grade?

As well as the procedures set up by an individual course to assess professional practice, there may be influence from the validating and/or professional body, as well as registration bodies, regarding the form and content of the final assessment. One of the requirements may be that a percentage of a year's cohort of students is examined by an external examiner. This mirrors what is done in written examination situations, where external examiners are appointed to monitor, and if necessary moderate the standard. When an external examiner reads a student's script it is painless for the student. Unfortunately, they will be only too aware if they are being observed in clinic by an external examiner! This situation is clearly very stressful for the student, and quite possibly for the clinical teacher too. It would seem to be wise to try to avoid it. Here, there is considerable need for maturity; those who have been set up by the profession in judgment of others need to exercise trust. It is really up to the individual course to ensure that clinical teachers are well prepared and supported in all aspects of their role, including that of assessment.

OTHER ASSESSMENTS RELATED TO WORK EXPERIENCE

An oral examination

In some instances a practical exam/assessment is followed by an oral (viva) for the purpose of discussing what went on in the practical situation and its relationship to the knowledge base. This procedure places considerable pressure on the student and may be influenced, rightly or wrongly, by the way the student is able to cope with the actual situation. There is some evidence that examiners are more lenient in the face-to-face situation (Cox, 1988). It is necessary to identify and evaluate the exact purpose of the oral examination carefully. It may in fact be attempting to assess something which can be assessed more appropriately in some other way. The oral/viva seems to be frequently used in health care courses, however it does have a number of drawbacks. For it to be equal all students would need to have seen/treated the same patient. This is almost impossible to arrange other than through observation of a video-recording, although 'judges differ in their assessment even when presented with identical evidence. Performances differ, even when students/doctors deal successfully with identical patients and problems' (Cox, 1988, p. 185).

Log books and diaries

The use of diaries and log books was introduced in Chapter 2 and later was raised in the context of introducing students to management skills, in Chapter 6. A report in the form of a **diary** appears to be a frequently used medium for providing a record of the placement experience, including patients seen/treated, locations, procedures undertaken, etc. Although this record is of some value, it can remain at a rather superficial descriptive level. The frequency with which the record is made varies with its purpose and the nature of the placement. Although some students may include an evaluative element.

The **log book** should not be so much like a diary format, but should give the opportunity for a deeper, more evaluative record of aspects of the work experience. It can form the basis of discussion either with the clinical teacher, college tutor or other students in clinic or in debriefing sessions back in college. The log book should emphasize the learning experiences generated through what has taken place, rather than just provide a record. It may focus on different aspects according to the aims of a particular placement, organization of the service or department; community work; describing and evaluating treatment planning and implementation; recording differences between patients with the same condition. It may also include personal reflection on the student's progress and professional development and could therefore include personal aims and objectives, and the methods of achieving them. It could also include evaluative comments on the way professionals work and the methods of teaching. It is in these areas that the development of the log book as a learning experience comes into conflict with its use as an assessment tool.

Reflection on some of these areas will be of immense value in learning, but students will be inhibited from including them if the log book forms part of their assessment and has to be handed in and shown to tutors. Log books which are handed in also covertly provide feedback information about the nature and quality of the placement to the institution. It is also necessary to know if external examiners have access to such material as log books and diaries.

Although log books are now being used more and more as part of the clinical assessment, care needs to be taken that their considerable learning potential is not devalued because it is also used for assessment.

Projects

Many courses, particularly those at degree level, require the student to undertake a project. This may be a literature review with a projected research plan, but may include a small empirical study with data collection and analysis, undertaken during the work experience. If the project is viewed by the institution as a substantial and important academic piece of work there may be considerable pressure on the student. The difficulties may be exacerbated where students are having their projects supervised by non-clinical teaching staff wishing to see their discipline developed to a high level by the students they supervise. If the project is ongoing during the period of the work experience there may be unfortunate repercussions on professional clinical progress, both because of the time and energy involved in data collection and the need to read extensively for the project, which is likely to be in a tightly-defined, specialist area. This may detract from clinically-related reading covering a wider spectrum. It is important that clinical teachers, students and all staff involved in project supervision, are helped to understand thoroughly the nature and status of the project, as they will then be able to judge how much it should impinge on the student's time. The weighting of marks between clinical work and project work needs to be considered.

In spite of the difficulties in projects they are nevertheless a valuable form of learning, allowing the student to pursue individual interests and strengths. Tomkins and McGraw (1988), say that 'student designed projects have demonstrated innovation that bring new perspectives to nursing practice and immeasurable rewards and satisfaction for both learners and teachers' (p. 179); this finding would be true for all health courses.

Case reports and case studies

Closely related to work with patients is the preparation of case reports or case studies. The difference between the two is not always easy to identify in course requirements. The **case report** appears to be much more like the 'real thing', that is, presenting case data and analysis in much the same way as would be done in clinical practice; it is very specific to an individual case.

The **case study** tends to require more theoretical discussion, going into the background of the nature and cause of a condition on which the diagnosis is based and the knowledge-base for the management and treatment selected, if possible referring to studies on the efficacy of particular treatment approaches.

Both the report and the study appear to provide a valuable learning experience for the student as they emphasize the need to reflect on the knowledge-base as it relates to clinical practice. The student who is weak at the basic knowledge level will have to work hard to produce a satisfactory report or study. Examples of the possible aims and purpose of the case study are shown in Box 8.7.

Box 8.7 Aims for case studies in two degree programmes

(a) BSc (Hons) in Occupational Therapy, Coventry Polytechnic

Through the case study the student will be given opportunity to:

1. consider in depth the difficulties being experienced by a selected patient/client;
2. identify the service being offered to the patient by the occupational therapist, and its significance in the overall care package/treatment regimen;
3. recognize the constraints imposed on that service;
4. evaluate the effectiveness of the service on the well-being of the patient/client;
5. consider ways in which the effectiveness may be enhanced.

(b) BSc Speech Pathology and Therapy, Leicester Polytechnic

The purpose of the case study is:

1. to develop your abilities to collect and collate data, appropriate to a particular patient;
2. to interpret the data colected;
3. to formulate managment aims, procedures and rationale;
4. to record events in therapy;
5. to evaluate the outcome of treatment and outline a tentative prognosis.

WHAT IS CLINICAL COMPETENCE TO BE JUDGED AGAINST?

Having decided which competencies we wish to make a judgement about it is then necessary to decide the standard against which the measure will be made. In a **norm referenced** procedure, the standard attributed to the performance of a student is a function of that performance in relation to that of other comparable students. In considering clinical competence it is difficult to decide who the comparable students are. Is it just the year group of that specific course in that year, or does it also relate to previous years? Does it relate further to students following similar professional courses in other institutions? Even with the use of external examiners, establishing some parity of standard is a difficult task.

The parity of standard across students from different institutions is of major importance, where on qualification, students are going to enter an identified field of practice. A more appropriate measure would be **criteria referenced**. In this type of assesment the standard to be reached is measured against some pre-specified criteria. (The driving test is another example of a criteria referenced test). There may of course be difficulties in agreeing the criteria, which need to be related to clinical competencies. The lists in Boxes 8.4 and 8.5 are examples of criteria. At the beginning of the chapter there was evidence that practitioners were able and willing to say what they would expect of a new practitioner. These criteria provide a good starting point. It is, however, difficult to define how specific the criteria need be. This is of major importance when practitioners enter fields in which the physical and psychological welfare of others is involved.

Institutions frequently require that a mark is provided for all pieces of assessment, including the assessment of work experience. Saxton and Ashworth (1990) hold that 'quantitative assessment of placement performance is wholly inappropriate'; they give several reasons, including; placements are not comparable; assessment gives more weight to the tangible elements of the job, neglecting such areas as motivation and attitudes ('motivational dispositions'), assessment affects and is affected by the students relationship with the placement teacher, etc. One must add to the incomparability of placements the difficulties of providing patients of equal difficulty and complexity. If institutions insist on a mark, how is this then to be arrived at? It is not too difficult to provide a mark for such elements as the log book and case books, etc. In my experience, clinicians feel extremely uncomfortable at being asked to assign a mark for the student's professional practice. They may find, however, that they are happier at identifying a letter grade, related to concepts of standards, such as the following:

A. Excellent/outstanding in all the elements of competence.
B. Well above average in all elements.
C. Acceptable performance in all elements of competence.
D. Acceptable in 2 out of 3 of the elements, but shows weakness in the third.
E. All elements are weak but show potential.
F. All elements lacking in development, lacks potential.

It is possible to assign marks to each of the letter grades:

A. 70% and above
B. 60–69%
C. 50–59%

D. 40–49%
E. 30–39%
F. 30 and below

Opportunities for resit should be very carefully considered with an F grade result. It can be seen that there is a close relationship between the grades and marks, with only ten points to each letter grade. In converting the letter grade to the mark, discussion between the clinical teacher and the college tutor would be valuable, to arrive at a more precise mark within the ten point band. The college tutor brings a wider experience of assessment as well as concepts of parity across students and perhaps courses.

WHY WOULD WE FAIL A STUDENT?

In the context of the above discussion it is useful to consider what we think would lead us to fail a student. Again, this is a topic which has been discussed by a number of clinical teachers. Like the expectations of the new entrant, clinical teachers do not hesitate in identifying the criteria they would use to judge a student as failing. Some of these are shown in Box 8.8.

Box 8.8 Criteria for failure: Multi-professional clinical teaching course, Yorkshire Health, 1991

(a) Physiotherapists

1. Ineffective/harmful.
2. Dangerous to patients, to profession and to image.
3. Poor attitudes and unacceptable attributes.
4. Inability to self-evaluate.
5. Inability to take advice and feedback and act on it to change behaviour.
6. Insensitivity to others.
7. Unwilling/incapable of improving performance despite all help offered.

(b) Speech and language therapists

1. Poor attendance.
2. Breaches of confidentiality.
3. Unable to take and maintain control.
4. Inability to self-evaluate.
5. Poor social/interpersonal skills.
6. Lack of content in therapy.
7. Inability to relate theory to practice.
8. Criminal record. Reference was made to the Code of Ethics and Professional Conduct, set up by the professional body.

Illott (1990) researched the problem of failing students in occupational therapy. Preliminary analysis of her data revealed the following criteria for failure:

- Lack of interpersonal skill
- Inappropriate attitudes
- Irresponsibility
- Breaches of confidentiality
- Failure to change or respond to feedback

It is interesting to compare these with the criteria listed in Boxes 8.8.

Although in theory we can list behaviours which would lead us to fail a student, in reality this may cause us considerable anguish. The difficulty of clinical teachers judging students they are working with, has been mentioned above. This difficulty arises not just because of the close and ongoing relationship between the student and the clinical teacher in the clinical setting, but may also be related to the view held by the teacher on the nature and role of being a teacher. Failing a student may be a particularly difficult task for the clinician who has a self-image of a caring and nurturing person (Meisenhelder, 1982; Illott, 1990). These feelings of the clinical teacher are exacerbated if the view of him/herself in the teaching role is one of being also responsible for the student's learning. The earlier discussion on an appropriate attitude to adult teaching and adult self-directed learning (androgogy), is of particular importance when it comes to final assessment of clinical competence. The process of adult learning has been interestingly discussed in the context of learning in occupational therapy students by Gaiptman and Anthony (1989). They stress the collaborative relationship between student and clinical teacher, which has implications for both the learning and assessment and evaluation process.

Throughout the student's learning through work experience, feedback should have been carried out in such a way that the student has a clear idea of his/her own abilities and weaknesses, having identified his/her own objectives and worked towards them. It therefore should not be that clinical teachers and college tutors are suddenly faced with making a decision about failing a student at the stage of the final assessment of clinical competence. Prior to this there will have been discussions with the staff and student regarding the student's standard and the likely assessment results. It is also essential that at the various stages of the course, clinical teachers and college tutors have not only provided clear feedback but have had the wisdom to fail a student if necessary. Illott (1990) believes that sometimes students are not failed because it is too painful for clinicians; seeing themselves as responsible for the student's learning, failing the student means that the clinical teacher has failed. It is also a temptation early on in the course to give the student the benefit of the doubt and to hope that the difficulties will be ironed out later on in the course. For some students, failing a stage of the course early on can have positive outcomes, either in establishng for them more clearly what they need to do to reach the required standard, or in helping them to consider a change of direction. It is clear that not only do students need help at a time of failure, but so also do the clinical teachers who are involved in reaching the decision.

This chapter has not set out to provide a prescription for clinical assessment. Rather it has tried to explore some of the important issues which need to be considered by all fields, in arriving at an assessment format.

FOLLOW-UP ACTIVITIES

1. Make a list of the competencies you would expect to be present in a newly qualified colleague coming to work in your department. (If you work in a specialist area make sure expectations are realistic for a new 'general practitioner'.) Compare your list with the lists found in Boxes 8.1, 8.2 and 8.3.
2. Obtain a course document from another field. Look in particular at the assessment of clinical practice. Evaluate the procedures used in the light of the issues discussed in this chapter.
3. Look at the criteria used for the assessment of competence in your own field. Do they include criteria for the three elements of competence – knowledge, skills and attitudes. Boxes 8.5, 8.6 and 8.7 give suggestions for the attitudes, knowledge and skill elements, which need to be assessed. You might like to prepare lists of criteria for all three elements of competence in your own field.
4. When you have listed the criteria ask yourself how easy/difficult it is to assess these and what might be the best method of doing so.

REFERENCES

Chatterton, D., Roberts, C. and Huston, F. (1988) *The Assessment of Supervised Work Experience*, Council for National Academic Awards.

Council for National Academic Awards (1989) *How Shall We Assess Them?* Information Service Discussion, Paper I.

Cox, K. (1988) How to Assess Performance, in Cox, K. and Ewan, E. (eds) *The Medical Teacher*, Churchill Livingstone, Edinburgh.

Caney, D. (1983) Competence – Can it be assessed? *Physiotherapy*, **69**, no. 8, 302–4.

Cross, V. (1992) Clinicians' Needs in Clinical Education: a report on a needs analysis workshop (in press).

Gaiptman, B. and Anthony, A. (1989) Contracting in Fieldwork Education: The model of Self-directed Learning. *Canadian Journal of Occupational Therapy*, **56**, no. 1, 10–14.

Helmer, O. (1964) *Convergence of Expert Concensus Through Feedback*. Paper 2973, Rand Corporation, Santa Monica, CA.

Heron, J. (1988) Assessment Revisited, in Boud, D. (ed.) *Developing Student Autonomy in Learning*, 2nd edn, Kogan Page, London; Nichols Publishing Co., New York.

Illott, I. (1990) Facing up to Failure. *Therapy Weekly*, **17**, no. 10, 6.

Meisenhelder, J.B. (1982) Clinical Evaluation: an instructor's dilemma. *Nursing Outlook*, Jan, 348–51.

Saxton, J. and Ashworth P. (1990) Sandwich Placements and the Visiting Tutor. *Journal of Further and Higher Education*, **14**, no. 1, 31–50.

Schwab, J.J. (1969) The Practical: A Language for the Curriculum. *School Review*, November, 1–23.

Schwab, J.J. (1971) The Practical: Arts of Eclectic. *School Review*, August, 493–541.

Stackhouse, J. and Furnham, A. (1983) A Student Centred Approach to the Evaluation of Clinical Skills. *British Journal of Disorders of Communication*, **18**, no. 3, 171–81.

Tomkins, C. and McGraw, M.J. (1988) In Boud, D. (ed.) (1988) *Developing Student Autonomy in Learning*, Kogan Page, London; Nichols Publishing Co., New York.

9

Practical work experience: a review of the literature

Jennifer Eastwood and Jane Whitehouse

INTRODUCTION

There is a vast amount of literature concerned with the nature and place of practice in formal education, with contributions from many fields including education, health care, business, engineering and science. Supervised work experience (SWE) is the term used by the Council for National Academic Awards (CNAA) for the practical or work-based components of college curricula and will be used in this chapter. Many graduate and undergraduate courses in health care and other fields have SWE as an important component of the students' programme.

The assumption of this chapter is that SWE in health care education is by no means a special case and that there is much to be gained from looking outside one's own field in order to clarify the principles involved. Many health care courses are now in the main stream of higher education and students and staff are consequently subjected to the same academic and environmental influences as students from non-health disciplines.

The term SWE implies that students are monitored or supervised during their practical placements. In health care courses this monitoring is invariably done by the college staff as well as by staff in the host institution. In other courses, such as business or science, the college may have less responsibility than the employer or host for supervision of students' work. Within health care courses themselves there is a range of work experience offered with placements ranging from blocks of practice, such as in sandwich courses, to attendance on a weekly basis concurrent with college attendance.

The literature which addresses these issues is variable in terms of content and style, and ranges from anecdotal or personal viewpoints to carefully designed and controlled research and experimentation. The following review, therefore, is a broad representation of the literature relating to SWE from many fields of study.

BENEFITS OF WORK EXPERIENCE

Sandwich education refers to the incorporation of a period of practical work experience into the educational course curriculum. Sandwich courses are offered in many disciplines, and, while the period of time students spend on placements may vary, successful completion of the practical component of the course is usually a requirement for qualification. The giant task of evaluating sandwich education overall has generally fallen to public bodies, with the conclusions of such evaluations being general rather than specific to a discipline or field.

The committee of Research into Sandwich Education (RISE) was set up by the Department of Education and Science in the UK to evaluate the available research on provision and effectiveness of sandwich courses across all disciplines. The RISE report (1985) concludes that, while few research studies control for differences between full-time and sandwich student populations, certain inferences about the outcomes of sandwich placements may still be drawn. Employers gain worthwhile benefits from sponsoring student placements with the gained value being greater than the overheads of salaries and other costs. While the majority of employers express no preference between sandwich graduates and graduates from courses without work experience, a significant minority of employers perceive benefits from the permanent recruitment of sandwich trained graduates in terms of a range of relevant skills. The RISE report also notes that the work entailed in the provision of sandwich courses encourages mutually beneficial links between higher education and industry.

The RISE committee recommends several courses of action if sandwich education is to continue to be advantageous to students and affordable for employers and colleges. A more critical attitude to sandwich placements should be adopted to ensure that placements are suitable, and to obviate the costs entailed in placing students in unsatisfactory work situations. The committee sugests that, where there is a shortage of good placements, colleges should not resign themselves to using unsatisfactory ones, but should endeavour to increase the numbers of placements provided by those which show a real commitment to sandwich education.

The RISE committee also recommends that colleges and employers make a concerted effort to secure the closest practicable relationship between the academic course content and the SWE. There is also a need for a greater awareness on the part of employers of the potential benefits to them of sandwich placements and for increased willingness to offer suitable placements to students.

The question of exactly how SWE benefits students' learning and in what ways this may be enhanced was found to be more difficult to address. The committee endorsed the need to evaluate the mechanisms by which SWE placements assisted student learning, but an analysis of this question was outside the committee's brief.

ARE PRACTICAL PLACEMENTS REALLY NECESSARY?

The CNAA appraisal of SWE in first degree courses (1984) reports the views of college staff on the values of placements in terms of costs, availability and success. The views of 96% of course leaders from CNAA sandwich courses were sampled. Eighty seven percent thought that the total learning currently achieved on the degree programme could not be achieved without the placement; 1% did not know, and 12% felt that it could. The latter view was predominantly made up of engineering and technology course leaders, and the majority of these did regard some simulated or practical experience as being necessary.

Course leaders also assessed personal and intellectual development, practical applications and skills' development as areas where SWE significantly contributed to students' educational progress. Placement provision and supervision by college tutors was found to be organized with reasonable economy, and direct benefits to employers were identified as being extensive, ranging from the opportunity to assess future employees to the fresh ideas which students may bring to the workplace.

The report raises some policy issues on the basis of the research findings. There was found to be considerable orthodoxy and conformity in the design of courses with SWE. The report notes that college staff appear to be willing to consider alternative patterns and modes of practical training, and suggests that this flexibility may be useful in a climate of reduced training budgets and facilities in all sectors.

As for the RISE report, the CNAA review skirts the educational implications of SWE as a part of students' learning experience and the ways in which these implications could be evaluated. The placement experiences of students on any course which involves SWE are considered generally to be worthwhile, but their place in the overall curriculum seems uncertain.

WORK EXPERIENCE AS PART OF THE CURRICULUM

The relationship of SWE or other types of practical education to theoretical, college-based learning is touched on in much of the literature in education. In the field of medical education, Harden (1986a) outlines some general issues which should be considered when planning curricula which include a practical component. These include consideration of the overall aims of the training programme, the learning methods which students will employ and the sequencing of the subject matter to be taught. These areas represent departures from the traditional narrow view of the curriculum which may have included only content and assessment of the course. Coles and Grant (1985) stress the need to integrate the practical learning which students will undertake into the curriculum rather than including experiential learning as a simple addition to lectures.

Harden (1986b) also discusses approaches to curriculum planning in the context of such factors as the rapidly developing knowledge-base and consumer pressure. Harden suggests that teachers should study the approaches to curriculum development which may be operating within their department. He outlines the characteristics of various approaches to the business of developing a curriculum such as the Aims and Objectives (engineering approach), Content (cookbook approach), Timetable (railway approach), Sponsorship (public relations approach) and the unrecommended 'magician' approach where it is not clear how the curriculum is developed. Harden emphasizes the need for consideration of the advantages and disadvantages of whatever approach to curriculum design is adopted.

The 'people's congress' approach to curriculum design is described by Harden as involving all the people who are contributing in any way to teaching the programme, including those who will contribute to students' practical experiences. Eliciting such a wide input is a time-consuming but potentially rewarding activity, facilitating curriculum change and being perceived by participants as more democratic than other approaches.

Some of Harden's suggestions may be applicable to curricula in SWE courses, particularly in view of the RISE recommendation that tutors should ensure the maximum relationship between practical and theoretical learning. This may be achieved in part through consideration of the methods of curriculum design. Studies which directly address the issue of the planning and development of curricula which include a large practical component are few, in spite of SWE being an important aspect of most health care and many other courses. The relationship of theoretical and practical education in courses containing SWE would seem to be a central issue for tutors and course leaders if SWE is to continue to be a major component of the course.

EVALUATING THE CURRICULUM

Once the curriculum is planned, its continued evaluation is seen as a central concern by a number of authors. Coles and Grant (1985) describe curriculum evaluation as the gathering of information about an educational programme for the purpose of making judgements about its merits. They state that, for any complex educational event such as SWE, there should be systematic qualitative and quantitative data collection, analysis and interpretation by all those involved in the programme in order for genuine educational development to occur. They also point out that the curriculum on paper may not be identical to the curriculum in action and that students' actual experiences of educational events may add yet another dimension to the situation. Where part of the curriculum involves practical experiences for individual students, the problem of identification and integration of these experiences becomes considerable.

Although, in many cases, SWE is an integral part of the curriculum, college staff may have relatively little control over the actual experiences students have on placements. The educational implications of this cannot be discounted, and studies which look at the benefits or otherwise of controlled or serendipitous practical experiences would be a welcome addition to the literature in this field.

It should be noted that Coles and Grant (1985) emphasize that changes based on the findings of curriculum evaluation may be difficult. Evaluation may provide information which the people concerned find unpalatable, and only superficial 'cosmetic' changes may be effected. However, careful reporting of the results of evaluation and involvement of the people concerned in all stages of the process should contribute greatly toward the implementation of educational development within the programme. Whether college staff would welcome the input of employers and placement supervisors into curriculum planning is a moot point; however, it must be acknowledged that, whether or not their contribution is actively sought, supervision of students on placements involves employers in educational events of considerable importance for the students who are placed with them.

TEACHING METHODS

From the field of medical education, Harden *et al* (1984) outline a model of curriculum analysis which can be used to tackle problems relating to the curriculum and to provide guidance regarding teaching methods and assessment. The model comprises six approaches to learning and teaching;

- Student-centred
- Problem-based
- Integrated
- Community-based
- Elective
- Systematic

It is called the SPICES model from the six initial letters of the names of the approaches.

Student-centred courses

In student-centred courses, Harden *et al.* (1984) state that students take much of the responsibility for their own learning and the emphasis of the course is on students and on what and how they learn. This contrasts with the more traditional teacher-centred model where the emphasis is on the formal lecture with the student being a passive recipient of knowledge. This was raised in Chapter 2, when teaching methods were reviewed. The problem-based aspect of courses refers to the emphasis on students solving 'real life' problems for which they must draw upon or acquire knowledge pertinent to the problem presented. Students may be given research problems, patient care problems or health delivery problems, contrasting in approach to courses which expect the student to engage in information gathering for its own sake as part of the development of a theoretical knowledge base. Student-centred approaches are of particular importance for adult learners who are preparing to become independent professionals responsible for providing health care.

Integrated teaching

Integrated teaching contrasts with discipline-based teaching and Harden *et al.* (1984) claim that integration reduces the fragmentation of traditional courses and allows students to perceive their discipline as a whole from an early stage. The community basis of the SPICES model contrasts with the hospital-based 'ivory tower' approach of older medical courses and is claimed to promote community orientation and to make use of the community for useful learning experiences for students. The development of electives as opposed to the standard, prescribed programme of subjects allows freedom within often overcrowded curricula, encourages students to take increased responsibility for their own learning and may facilitate career choice by allowing students to explore their interest in a particular area.

Systematic or planned learning approaches contrast with the apprenticeship or opportunistic programme still employed in many medical and other health-related courses. These approaches reflect the belief that what students do and see should no longer be left to chance but should be both planned and recorded. Harden *et al.* (1984) state that this view is part of a trend toward more accountability, where the public and educational authorities may require assurances about the products of medical schools and other institutions educating health personnel.

Essential learning

While Harden *et al.* (1984) present contrasting extremes of style in curriculum analysis, their work raises several issues for course planners involved in the development of practical experiential education in whatever discipline. Is SWE inherently student-centred, and, if so, does this contribute to its success? Are work experiences basically problem-solving exercises for students in which they may learn to apply their theoretical knowledge? Unlike many college tutors, employers' expertise may seldom reflect a narrow discipline area, thereby encouraging integration of their students' knowledge. Placements in the health service, business and commerce may have a much closer relationship to the community than has the training school or college. Does SWE expose students to this community orientation, thereby enabling them to see their learning in context?

Learning styles

Implicit in the evaluation of curriculum is the idea of how and why students learn. The implications of the learning styles which students may adopt have been evaluated by Newble and Entwistle (1986) and relate to practical and theoretical education in a number of fields. The authors divide students' learning into two main approaches; the surface approach, which is based on rote learning and memorization of pieces of information, and the deep approach which is characterized by the intention to understand the material or subject and to relate this understanding to the student's own experience and previous knowledge. Newble and Entwistle state that teaching styles and curricula may facilitate one or the other approach, often without the awareness of tutors involved, and that certain types of assessment may in fact hinder the deep approach to learning which most schools would wish to encourage.

The role of practical experience in facilitating the deep approach to learning in students is a question which may profitably be addressed by future research. For tutors and course leaders involved in curriculum design and assessment in courses where SWE is a component, the issues raised by Harden *et al.* and Newble and Entwistle may have numerous applications.

The diversity of curriculum issues addressed in the literature from the field of medical education contrasts strongly with studies from other fields where practical education is also important. The question of whether practical and project work are central or peripheral to courses in engineering is addressed by Cornwall (1975) who states that traditional didactic approaches to teaching are inappropriate to the education of engineers. Cornwall pleads for practical work to form the orientation, rather than just one element of science-based courses. Waite (1982), however, suggests that budgetary cutbacks in both public and private training allowances are likely to limit, at least for the time being, the increased integration of practical elements into many courses.

An integrated practical and college-based curriculum may not necessarily be a more expensive option. Mennin and Martinez-Burrola (1986) found that the costs of a traditional and a problem-based curriculum were identical. Many of the issues raised in the literature on curricula indicate a reorganization rather than a reallocation or increase of resources. The financial rather than the educational implications of SWE are at issue in much of the literature. What the student on placement actually learns is, however, an important and relevant aspect of research.

THE NATURE AND OUTCOMES OF EXPERIENTIAL LEARNING

The nature of the learning which takes place in SWE and other types of practical education has been discussed by several authors, and, given the importance of practical education in many courses, the question or whether cognitive knowledge is acquired through practical experience or whether the outcomes of such experience are in some way different to those of traditional classroom teaching methods is central to any review.

Jones, Cason and Cason (1986) found that medical students attending clinics scored no better on tests of those areas where they had had clinical experience than areas where their learning was purely theoretical. The authors suggest that several circumstances could explain this finding, however, including the variability of clinical experiences and the possibility that clinics may have been too busy to permit discussion of the students' experiences. While highlighting the likely alternative benefits of practical experience, such as change in attitudes and problem-solving ability, Jones *et al.* point out the need for clear delineation of the goals of the curriculum and state that such goals may not, in fact, include an increase in cognitive or theoretical knowledge.

Mayo and Jones (1985), however, state that differences were apparent in civil engineering student degree classifications depending on whether the students were on a straight 3-year degree or a 4-year sandwich degree. There were no reported differences between the two groups and both received the same lectures, but the sandwich students overall received higher-classed degrees that the full-time students, regardless of A-level results. The reasons for this outcome are unknown, but may be related to personal observation of the workplace, maturation or stronger desire for employment.

The problems inherent in identification of what constitutes experiential learning are elaborated in the CNAA report on assessing prior experiential learning in mature students applying for admission to polytechnic courses (Evans, 1988). This report emphasizes that experience *per se* is not the same as the knowledge, skills and competencies which result from it, but that there is, as yet, no defined framework on which to assess the exact nature of the learning which occurs as a result of practical experience.

The early review of Ward and Webster (1965) questioned the nature of learning in speech therapy clinical training programmes. The authors cite the development of human qualities such as empathy and personal development as being as valid as specific professional skills and attitudes for students' acquisition in practical learning. The development of such qualities would presumably be a valid outcome of most health care courses.

Literature addressing the question of what is learned through experience is sparse; however, there is general agreement among authors that practical learning may involve inherently different qualities than formal, college-based learning. The concept of competence is one which is particularly relevant to SWE and practical learning and is one which appears worthy of further consideration and research and is of central concern in the education of health care professionals.

THE ACQUISITION OF SKILLS THROUGH WORK EXPERIENCE

There is little doubt that the acquisition of skills of various kinds is seen by all those involved as a beneficial outcome of SWE. Technical, interpersonal and specific communication skills may all be expected to be developed to some extent in the context of practical experience. Whether these skills are the focus of formal training preliminary to the experience, or whether they are acquired incidentally to other outcomes of placements, is a question which has been addressed by several authors.

Bleys *et al.* (1986) used self-assessment by students to bridge the gap between theoretical study and practical experience in medical school and found that prior experience within the health care system appeared to have a positive effect on skill acquisition. They suggest that early active experience of health care in the curriculum fosters the development of practical skills as well as insight into the relevance of theoretical studies. Black and Harden (1986) suggest that skills such as interviewing and case history taking may be developed by providing feedback to medical students during, rather than after practical examinations. The use of feedback to help student learning has been thoroughly discussed in Chapter 7 of this volume.

Tidmarsh (1984) describes the difficulties of getting social work students to apply skills learned in specific skills' training sessions to their practical casework. Students claimed that application of formally learned skills felt artificial, although the act of engaging in the casework itself did not. Interviews with the students revealed that some feared that using formally-trained skills would take away their valued sense of relationship with their clients. Tidmarsh overcame this 'artificiality barrier' by highlighting for students one of the aims of social work education: to develop a practitioner who can use skills consistently within the context of relationship. The fostering of trust and provision of sensitive feeback for students facilitated their acceptance of this model of working.

As cited in the CNAA Training Uses of Placement Research Report (1983), engineering and business studies sandwich courses students were asked for their views regarding the development of three sets of skills on placement; interpersonal, technical and applicatory skills. The consensus in both disciplines was that interpersonal skills were the most greatly developed by placements. Engineers felt that technical and applicatory skills were developed on placement to a greater extent than did those involved in business studies courses. Despite these findings, both groups stated that task-orientated skills should be considered more important for development on a placement than people oriented skills.

The development of interpersonal skills

Despite the opinion that interpersonal skills constitute the group of skills most frequently developed in practice, the CNAA Goals of Engineering Education report (Beuret and Webb, 1983) suggests that high percentages of engineers and their colleagues consider the engineers' ability to 'express and communicate both verbally and in writing' is 'a problem'. This report suggests engineers tend to lack the human and social skills their jobs require, and yet when listing the most important abilities their jobs demanded, engineers rated technical skills, communications and human relationships as first, second and third.

Hargie and Morrow (1985) define competence in many types of profession as involving the ability to execute three main sets of skills:

- Cognitive skills: the knowledge base of the profession
- Technical or psychomotor skills: manipulative skills inherent within the tasks performed
- Social or communication skills: ability to interact effectively with others

(These are very like the three elements of competence; knowledge, skills and attitudes, considered in the model of practice in Chapter 1.) While traditional education and training of most professional groups has placed emphasis on the first two at the expense of the latter, Hargie and Morrow cite Ellis and Whittington's (1981) claim that most occupations demand interaction with others at times and some jobs have skilled interaction as a primary focus. These jobs include the 'interpersonal' professions such as counsellors, teachers, social workers, paramedical and medical personnel, sales people and managers. This point was raised earlier in the context of providing clinical teaching courses to different professional groups.

Research in medical education has addressed the topic of the skills required for effective communication with patients. Burnett and Thompson (1986) describe a successful attempt to raise the level of medical students' understanding of patients' lifestyles and medical knowledge and Knox and Bouchier (1985) outline an introductory course in teaching communication skills to pre-clinical medical students. Alroy, Ber and Kramer's (1984) evaluation of the short-term effects of an interpersonal skills course for such students using videotaped trigger films and discussion, showed that the group demonstrated a significant increase in caring activitiy, kindness and self-confidence while a control group were observed to go through the 'dehumanization' process often reported in the medical literature, showing significant reductions in caring, kindness and respect for the patient.

Hargie and Morrow (1985) describe how communication skills' training is incorporated into the undergraduate education of pharmacists in the United States, but not in the UK. Their paper outlines a short microtraining course in communication skills as part of a continuing education programme for pharmacists in the UK, and claims that this is the first documented report of such training for pharmacists in the UK. The course provides what Ellis and Whittington (1981) call Specialist Social Skills Training (SSST) and is designed for professionals who have achieved 'at least normal levels of skill but who have particular vocational or professional objectives which necessitate sophisticated or specialised forms of interaction'.

The idea that SSST course needs will not necessarily be the same across different professional groups is mentioned by Saunders and Caves (1986). Their paper summarizes attempts to identify specific clinical skills used by speech therapists, and reveals how speech therapists may use certain skills such as encouragement, questioning and building rapport in a highly differentiated fashion compared to other professionals. Klevans, Voltz and Friedman (1981) trained speech therapy undergraduates in interpersonal communication skills and found that those participating in an experiential programme used more verbal facilitative responses in the initial stages of a helping relationship, than did those students who participated in a theoretical programme. Other health care workers may also need to use social skills in highly specialized ways.

The work of Haynes and Oratio (1978) and Oratio (1976, 1978) indicates that speech therapy students, supervisors and clients share the perception that professional or technical skills and interpersonal skills are central components of practical competence. The central importance of interpersonal skills in several of the health care professions was noted earlier. Outstanding student clinicians tend to receive the highest grades on all clinical skills (Dowling, 1985), but it should be noted that almost all students receive good grades from their supervisors. This may imply that practical training is more effective than academic training, or perhaps that supervisors are too lenient in judging clinical skills.

When is it best to learn skills?

On the basis of the literature, it is difficult to assess whether skills considered important in the workplace are best learned through practical experience on the job or by means of specific skills' training which could take place at college. When considering the subject of skills' training as part of professional education in the human services disciplines, it may be relevant to consider the paradox revealed by Cole and Lacefield (1978). Skill domains which go well beyond the usual intellective and cognitive professional–technical requirements, and are considered vital to effective practice, may also be considered less possible and appropriate to teach and evaluate, regardless of the educational setting.

ATTITUDES AND CHARACTERISTICS OF PARTICIPANTS IN SWE

There are three main groups of participants in work experience: students, their clinical teachers/supervisors/employers and college tutors. The perceptions and attitudes of these participants have been evaluated in several studies.

Students' perceptions

Kautzmann (1987) identifies several differences in the perceptions of occupational therapy students and supervisors with regard to the purposes of initial practical fieldwork. Students were concerned that their fieldwork should give them an opportunity to learn the specific skills of clinical practice, while their supervisors valued broader outcomes of fieldwork such as the development of awareness of the patient as a whole person. Kautzmann suggests that supervisors should be aware of these differences between their own and students' primary objectives and should implement specific teaching to enable students to expand their expectations.

Smith (1985) describes the attitudes of applied physics undergraduates on a sandwich course to their year of professional training. Students were placed in government and commercial research laboratories, productions works and bioengineering centres and were canvassed on:

1. amount of help and advice given during the placement;
2. the value they placed on the experience;
3. degree of integration of practical and theoretical work;
4. impact on final-year projects and choice of career.

Students broadly agreed that their placements were worthwhile, but felt that their preparation from college staff was inadequate. Students felt that the quality of practical training itself was good from the viewpoints of relevance, intellectual demand and modern applications. There was a varied response on the question of the degree to which the practical experience had integrated with college course-work, and a general agreement that the visits from college tutors during the placement were not as helpful as students might wish them to be. The nature and objectives of such visits was fully explored in Chapter 7 of this volume.

Daniel and Pugh (1975) looked at the attitudes of business studies' students and their employers to their sandwich year. They concluded that while the respondents perceived the quality of industrial placements on the whole to be reasonable, the level of integration between the sandwich year and the academic course content was less satisfactory. Tutors' visits to students during their sandwich placements were generally viewed as inadequate.

Dowling and Wittkop (1982) found that speech therapy students' perceptions of supervision practices on their practical training differed significantly according to the time they had spent on the placements and the site where their practical training took place. The authors reflect that this variability may indicate that students generally accept unquestioningly the amount and style of supervision offered on their particular placement, and that they have few standards of what supervision should entail or how it should be conducted. Students tended to accept and adopt the standards of their practice placement supervisor, although their identification of their needs for supervision did alter (although not reduce) with increased experience.

College tutors' perceptions

Day *et al.* (1982) outline what they, as college tutors, see as the benefits of sandwich courses in business studies. These include the development of student insight into the relationship between theory and practice, the experience of working with others, the opportunity for the student to mature and accept responsibility and the chance for the student to 'test the water' of his or her chosen career.

Horne's (1980) assessment of the value of sandwich education in quantity surveying is based on the assumption that careful preparation and observation of students by college staff must inevitably lead to a beneficial experience for both student and sponsor. While this assumption may not be entirely unfounded, the studies of Smith (1985) and Jones *et al.* (1986) illuminate the need for evaluation of the specific outcomes of placements and suggest that the perceived satisfaction of college tutors and employers may not be an adequate measure of the placement's effectiveness.

Characteristics of fieldwork teachers

The characteristics of those individuals who supervise students during their practical work have been studied by several authors. Anderson (1981) stresses the need for specialized training of supervisors/clinical teachers to enable them to adopt a variety of teaching styles and to establish the best supervisor–supervisee relationships. The need for the development of courses for clinical teachers working with health care students is central to the ideas explored in this book.

Crago and Pickering (1987) comprehensively review the teaching, professional and interpersonal aspects of supervising students on clinical placements (in speech therapy) and conclude that the role and responsibilities of supervisors are unique, requiring self-exploration and accurate perceptions of interpersonal dynamics by the effective supervisor. Models of supervision relevant to health care disciplines are outlined by Oratio (1977) who states that the supervision process may be student-centred, supervisor-centred or patient-centred, with each style having advantages and disadvantages for all parties. The role and responsibilities of the clinical teacher was fully explored in Chapter 3.

EMPLOYMENT PROSPECTS

Bourner's (1982) study of the relationship between sandwich placements and the employment of polytechnic business studies graduates concludes that placements enhance the students' prospects, and, interestingly, reduce their perceived needs for further full-time study. Bourner also notes that sandwich placements encourage students to enter manufacturing industry rather than the educational sector, public service or commerce in spite of the more attractive salaries and status of the latter.

The place of sandwich education in determining the student's future employment has been evaluated by much of the literature on cooperative education. McRobbie (1985) includes the advantages of selection of future employees among the benefits received by a small firm from the sponsorship of sandwich students. Wright (1985) endorses this view and also believes that training programmes should be agreed between tutors and placement supervisors and that student progress should be monitored by exchanging visits.

IS SWE EFFECTIVE?

The CNA Training Instruments Pack (TIP, Dorsman, 1984) is specifically designed to test the relevance and effectiveness of SWE and thereby to enhance its quality for all participants. It comprises three parts; college staff guidelines, the training objectives profiles and the market needs' survey. It is the result of research carried out at five polytechnics and colleges throughout the UK. Twelve courses in total were involved. Seven of these were business studies and related courses and five were engineering courses.

The methodology behind the development of the TIP is outlined in the CNAA Training uses of Placement Research Report (1983). Views regarding quality, effectiveness and relevance of SWE were collected from students, college staff and employers by means of questionnaires and interviews. All data were subject to factor analysis and cross tabulation procedures using the Statistical Package for Social Sciences. The researchers found seven major factors were perceived as substantial training objectives by the respondents:

- Interpersonal and social skills
- Insight into the world of work
- Interrelationships of theory and practice
- Personal development
- Additional and indirect benefits of placements
- Career preparation
- Technical development

The resulting Training Objectives Profiles were designed to be used in a number of ways, including construction of personal profiles and comparison between individuals; matching individual students to employers and planning placement programmes; comparisons of students' aspirations and beliefs pre- and post-placement; and the creation of benchmark profiles of groups against which individuals can compare. The researchers claim that these applications should lead to resolution of some of the differences between the groups.

In an analysis of the use of the TIP, Dorsman (1984) states that the pack has been used in a variety of ways since its publication. Staff have used the TIP to encourage students to broaden their expectations of placement experiences and it has been instrumental in helping staff and employers to explore their different perceptions of the purposes of placements. The research which led to the development of the TIP has revealed that there is a broad set of factors in SWE which describe its content and against which individual objectives of participants may be measured. The importance placed upon these factors has been shown to vary amongst participants and, therefore, has highlighted the need for careful planning and evaluation of the process of SWE in any course in which it is a requirement.

A more recent CNAA funded project concerned an appraisal of SWE in speech therapy education (Shute *et al.*, 1989). The study was conducted across two speech therapy courses in the UK leading to a degree and a licence to practice; the 4-year honours degree at Birmingham Polytechnic comprising 'thin' sandwich mode SWE and the 3-year ordinary degree at Leicester

Polytechnic comprising concurrent mode SWE. Data were collected from students, clinical teachers and college tutors from both courses.

Analysis of the data revealed twelve factors which respondents thought to be of importance in effective SWE:

- Preparation for employment
- Getting through
- Professional competence
- Development of theory-based clinical practice
- General management skills
- Clinical management skills
- Independent decision-making
- Interpersonal and social skills
- Realistic work experience
- Other benefits of the education and health care services partnership
- Commitment to a career in speech therapy
- Clinical skills

Perceptions of the relative importance of these factors varied across the groups of respondents.

SOURCE MATERIALS FOR STUDENTS AND CLINICAL TEACHERS

Students may wish to develop a perspective on what is, in many cases, a new area of learning and teaching. Supervisors may need an overview of the clinical teaching process in an easily accessible form. For these people there are several handbooks and sources of information available.

McQuade and Graessle (1990) outline suggestions for making the most of work experience. Although primarily for secondary students, much of the content is relevant to work experience programmes at any stage in education and includes ideas for preparation of students, designing assignments while students are on placement, giving information to students, problem solving and points about how an equal opportunities policy may apply in the SWE setting.

Leith *et al.*'s (1989) supervision handbook offers a behavioural model on which to base information and activities concerning supervisor roles, evaluation strategies and identification and encouragement of specific student skills and behaviours. Watts (1990) presents a largely activity-based approach to clinical teaching which may form a useful introductory text for first-time clinical teachers. Watts covers a broad range of health care fields and offers interesting case study material on which to base the learning and teaching exercises.

Also of interest in this context is the paper by Hagler and Casey (1990) which addresses the games clinical teachers/supervisors play. It is written from the standpoint of the student. The authors suggest that the clinical teaching setting offers many opportunities for manipulation of one participant by another – usually of students by clinical teachers/supervisors. This manipulation may be understood in terms of games; for example, the game 'You're Doing Just Fine' may be a way of fobbing off problem students and, therefore, reducing supervisor responsibilities. The game 'I Wondered When You Would Figure That Out' allows supervisors to maintain face or image when confronted with a student who raises points which the supervisor had not thought of. The content, while offered in a spirit of fun, has serious implications for the clinical teaching process. Experienced supervisors may read this with some sense of uncomfortable familiarity.

SUMMARY AND CONCLUSIONS ON THE RESEARCH ON SWE

The research relating to experiential learning is widely variable in style, scope and design. This poses obvious difficulties for comparison of results. Considering the extent of the field to be covered in any evaluation of SWE, these discrepancies are probably not surprising.

The reports on the value of experiential learning in the workplace are almost universally positive from all authors in all disciplines. The consensus is that the experiences have value for students in numerous ways, although these are by no means yet clearly delineated. There are also benefits accruing to the institutions which provide placements, whether in business, health care or some other field, and positive benefits to the college or training school as well.

There are strong indications that curriculum planning must accommodate experiential learning in an integrated way and that course planners cannot hope to ensure beneficial experiential learning for students by merely attaching a practical placement onto an otherwise unmodified college curriculum. Inclusion of work experience requires creative and innovative curriculum design with the emphasis away from traditional discipline-based courses if all parties are to benefit.

The nature of the learning which takes place during SWE is poorly-defined. Competence and specific skills are obvious components of SWE educational outcomes, but much further research is required if this important issue is to be identified and developed. The assessment of students' work on placements by employers or college staff is a closely related issue, and until it can be identified that students are acquiring particular knowledge and skills on placements, the assessment of students must be, at best, inadequate.

Characteristics of the students, college tutors and work experience teachers who participate in SWE also assume importance in any evaluation of the effectiveness of the process. Individual perceptions, personalities and expectations are involved in this mode of learning and the qualities of participants and the ways such qualities may affect the outcomes of placements are little understood. The perceptions of participants as to what constitutes effective SWE are central to an understanding of experiential learning. It is hoped that the insight gained from looking at work experience from a number of different fields and perspectives will enhance the reader's understanding of some of the processes involved.

REFERENCES

Alroy, G., Ber, R. and Kramer, D. (1984) An evaluation of the short-term effects of an interpersonal skills course, *Medical Education*, **18**, no. 2, 85–9.

Anderson, J.L. (1981) Training of supervisors in speech–language pathology and audiology *American Speech and Hearing Association*, **23**, 77–82.

Beuret, G. and Webb, A. (1983) *Goals of Engineering Education (GEEP) Engineers – Servants or Saviours*, CNAA Development Services Publication 2, London.

Black, N.M.I., and Harden, R.M. (1986) Providing feedback to students on clinical skills by using the Objective Structured Clinical Examination, *Medical Education*, **20**, no. 1, 48–52.

Bleys, C., Gerritsma, J.G.M. and Netjes, I. (1986) Skills development by medical students and the influence of prior experience: A study using evaluation by students and self assessment *Medical Education*, **20**, no. 5, 234–9.

Bourner, T. (1982) The impact of sandwich placement on the employment of polytechnic business studies graduates, *Bulletin of Education Research*, **23**, 32–46.

Burnett, A.C. and Thompson, D.G. (1986) Aiding the development of communication skills in medical students *Medical Education*, **20**, no. 5, 424–31.

Cole, H.P. and Lacefield, W.E. (1978) Skill domains critical to the helping professions, *Personnel and Guidance Journal*, Oct. 54–7.

Coles, C.R. and Grant, J. (1985) Curriculum evaluation in medical and health care education, *Medical Education*, **19**, 4, 405–22.

Cornwall, M.G. (1975) Sandwich education and project work: Do they have the same aims? *European Journal of Engineering Education*, **1**, Summer, 41–7.

Council for National Academic Awards (1983) *Training Uses of Placement; The Research Report*, CNAA Development Services, Paper 2, London.

Council for National Academic Awards (1984) *Supervised Work Experience in CNAA First Degree Courses: An Appraisal*, CNAA Development Services, Publication 5, London.

Crago, M.B. and Pickering, M. (1987) *Supervision in Human Communication Disorders*, Little, Brown and Co., Boston.

Daniel, W.W. and Pugh, N. (1975) *Sandwich Courses in Higher Education PEP Report on CNAA Degrees in Business Studies*, PEP Broadsheet no. 557.

Day, J., Kelly, M.J., Parker, D. and Farr, M.F. (1982) The role of industrial training in business studies sandwich degrees *Business Education*, Summer, 105–22.

Department of Education and Science (1985) *An Assessment of the Costs and Benefits of Sandwich Education*, Research into Sandwich Education Committee, GPB-5524, British Lending Library.

Dorsman, M. (1984) Experiential learning in undergraduate study. The Training Instruments Pack: an instrument for identifying and assessing the objectives of supervised work experience in educational courses, *Journal of Assessment and Evaluation in Higher Education*, **9**, no. 1, 57–61.

Dowling, S. (1985) Clinical performance characteristics of failing, average and outstanding clinicians, *The Clinical Supervisor*, **3**, no. 3, 49–54.

Dowling, S. and Wittkop, J. (1982) Students' perceived supervisory needs, *Journal of Communication Disorders*, **23**, 46–51.

Ellis, R. and Whittington, D. (1981) *A Guide to Social Skills Training*, Croom Helm, London.

Evans, N. (1988) *An Assessment of Prior Experiential Learning*, CNAA Development Services, Publication 17, London.

Hagler, P. and Casey, P. (1990) Games supervisors play in clinical supervision. *American Speech and Hearing Association*, **32**, 2, 53–6.

Harden, R.M., Sowden, S. and Dunn, W.R. (1984) Educational strategies in curriculum development; the SPICES model, *Medical Education*, **18**, no. 3, 284–97.

Harden, R.M. (1986a) Ten questions to ask when planning a curriculum, *Medical Education*, **20**, no. 4, 356–65.

Harden, R.M. (1986b) Approaches to curriculum planning, *Medical Education*, **20**, no. 5, 458–66.

Hargie, O. and Morrow, N. (1985) Interpersonal communication and professional practice; A case study from pharmacy, *Journal of Further and Higher Education*, **9**, no. 3, 26–39.

Haynes, W.O. and Oratio, A.R. (1978) A study of clients' perceptions of therapeutic effectiveness. *Journal of Speech and Hearing Disorders*, **43**, 21–3.

Horne, A. (1980) The role of sandwich training in professional education, *The Quantity Surveyor*, **36**, no. 9, 170–2.

Jones, J.G., Cason, G.J. and Cason, C. (1986) The acquisition of cognitive knowledge through clinical experiences, *Medical Education*, **20**, no. 1, 10–12.

Kautzmann, L. (1987) Perceptions of the purpose of level 1 fieldwork, *The American Journal of Occupational Therapy*, **41**, no. 9, 595–600.

Klevans, D.R., Voltz, H.B. and Friedman, R.M. (1981) A comparison of experiential and observational approaches for enhancing the interpersonal communication skills of speech–language pathology students, *Journal of Speech and Hearing Disorders*, **46**, no. 7, 203–13.

Knox, J.D.E. and Bouchier, I.A.D. (1985) Communication skills teaching, learning and assessment, *Medical Education*, **19**, no. 4, 285–9.

Leith, W., McNeice, E. and Fusilier, B. (1989) *Handbook of Supervision: A Cognitive-Behavioural System*, Little Brown and Co., Boston.

Mayo, R.H. and Jones, L.L. (1985) The effect of a sandwich year on degree classification, *Positive Partnerships. World Conference on Co-operative Education*, **2**, 428–31.

Mennin, S.P. and Martinez-Burrola, N. (1986) The cost of traditional medical education, *Medical Education*, **20**, no. 5, 187–94.

McRobbie, I.M. (1985) A small firm's view on co-operative education, *Positive Partnerships World Conference on Co-operative Education*, Conference Papers, **2**, 373–6.

McQuade, P. and Graessle, L. (1990) *Making the Most of Work Experience*, Cambridge University Press.

Newble, D.I. and Entwistle, N.J. (1986) Learning styles and approaches: implications for medical education, *Medical Education*, **20**, no. 5, 162–75.

Oratio, A.R. (1976) A factor analytic study of criteria for evaluating student clinicians in speech pathology, *Journal of Communication Disorders*, **9**, 199–210.

Oratio, A.R. (1977) *Supervision in Speech Pathology*, University Park Press, Baltimore.

Oratio, A.R. (1978) Comparative perceptions of therapeutic effectiveness by student clinicians and clinical supervisors, *American Speech and Hearing Association*, **20**, 959–62.

Saunders, C. and Caves, R. (1986) An empirical approach to the identification of communication skills with reference to speech therapy, *Journal of Further and Higher Education*, **10**, no. 2, 29–44.

Shute, C.T., Eastwood, J., Whitehouse, J. and Freeman, M. (1989) *An Appraisal of Supervised Work Experience in Speech Therapy Training*, Birmingham and Leicester Polytechnics.

Smith, E.V. (1985) An evaluation of the attitudes of sandwich course undergraduates in applied physics to their one year in professional training, *Journal of Further and Higher Education*, **9**, no. 1, 71–7.

Tidmarsh, C. (1984) Beyond the artificiality barrier: An exploration, *Social Work Education*, **4**, no. 1, 7–9.

Watts, N. (1990) *Handbook of Clinical Teaching*, Churchill Livingstone, London.

Waite, T. (1982) Sandwich courses, *Training Officer*, **18**, no. 5, 112–3.

Ward, L.M. and Webster, E.J. (1965) The learning of clinical competence skills in speech pathology, *American Speech and Hearing Association*, Feb, 38–40.

Wright, J.B. (1985) Negative elements in positive partnerships *Positive Partnerships*. *World Conference on Co-operative Education*, Conference Papers, Vol. 2, 377–9.

Appendix A: A revised model of the elements of professional competence*

SURFACE
⇅
1st DEEP LEVEL
	1. Techniques and procedures
	including skills in interpersonal relationships
	⇅
	2. Knowledge and understanding
	  2.1 Speech and language pathology knowledge
	  2.2 Linguistic knowledge
	  2.3 Psychological knowledge
	  2.4 Child development knowledge
	  2.5 Sociological knowledge
	  2.6 Clinical medicine knowledge
	  2.7 KNOWLEDGE AWARENESS
	⇅

2nd DEEP LEVEL
Giving meaning
to what is done
and influencing
use of knowledge,
techniques and
procedures.
	3. Attitudes
	  3.1 Relationships with clients/patients
	  3.2 Relationships with carers.
	  3.3 Relationships with other professionals.
	  3.4 Relationship with employer.
	  3.5 Planning and evaluation.
	  3.6 Professional work and career future.
	⇅
	4. Moral values

ALL LEVELS INFLUENCED BY:
  Life experiences
  Pre-registration learning
  Work experience
  Continuing education
  Relationship with employing authority
  Work context, e.g. hospital, school,
    clinic, private practice.

*Adapted from Stengelhofen (1984)

Index

Page numbers given in italic represent boxes, those in bold represent figures